THE LIVING R᎒ ᎒ᵣ ᎒ᵣᵤRY

Pioneering Mental Health Awareness in the Church

Marja Bergen

THE LIVING ROOM STORY:
Pioneering Mental Health Awareness in the Church

Copyright © 2020 Marja Bergen

All rights reserved. Neither this publication nor any part of this publication may be reproduced or transmitted in any form or by any means, electronic or mechanical, including photocopying, recording or any information storage and retrieval system, without permission in writing from the author.

Photography by Marja Bergen.
Cover art by Wes Bergen

All Scripture quotations, unless otherwise specified, are taken from the Holy Bible, New International Version®, NIV® Copyright ©1973, 1978, 1984, 2011 by Biblica, Inc.® Used by permission. All rights reserved worldwide. Holy Bible, New International Version. Used by permission. All rights reserved worldwide.

Marja Bergen
www.marjabergen.com

ACKNOWLEDGEMENTS

The years that followed the end of this story were difficult ones. I'm deeply grateful to those friends and acquaintances who continue supporting me. I have the love of many. If I tried to list you all, there would be a danger of leaving names out that should be included. Please know you're remembered in my mind.

I've been well looked after by the staff at Burnaby Hospital. So good to have both a psychiatrist to treat me and a case manager to help me with my day to day needs.

My therapist, Grant McMahon, has been a great friend—the most understanding person I've ever talked to. I must be his oldest client and I'm not about to leave him soon.

I'm grateful for my family, my son Cornelius and his wife Jeannette. Glad to have them living close by.

But most of all, I thank my husband Wes. I could never have lived the life I did without you by my side. Thank you for all you've been to me.

CONTENTS

CARRYING ON THE BATTLE

I dedicated over twenty years of my life to fighting the stigma of mental illness. As this book will show, I accomplished much. But in the end, I myself was hurt by stigma, causing serious damage to my mental health. Today, I recognize more than ever that the battle must continue.

I thank God for having given me the strength and determination to put this story together—this celebration of what was good and what brought me joy.

I pray that *The Living Room Story* will in some way become another building block to reduce the stigma that hurts so many.

Marja

INTRODUCTION

My years with *Living Room*, from the founding in 2006 to my retirement in 2015, were the best years of my life. Although I had many ups and downs during that time, I mostly remember how happy I was to serve the Lord in supporting people with mental health problems. I knew that this was what God made me to do.

At the time, there was little understanding about mental illness. People in church were hurt by ignorant comments that made them feel humiliated. They were blamed for their depression, made to feel it was caused by a poor relationship with God. For some, *Living Room* became like a church to many. Here they were assured they had nothing to be ashamed of.

I loved the members of my group. It felt good to walk with them through their trials, because I felt Jesus walking with us. After the group meetings I frequently had an indescribable feeling that could only be described as "holy joy."

Living Room members studied and discussed Scripture together. Through these studies, they learned to cope, survive, and even thrive. Bolstered by the knowledge of God's love, they were encouraged to trust him. They gathered the strength and confidence to face a world that did not understand them.

Members came to believe that no matter their health challenges or pain, God would not leave them alone with it. Jesus was with them. He understood what they were going through in a way the world never would.

With a love that came to them through Jesus, they buoyed each other up with reminders that God would help them overcome. *Living Room* members had an understanding not available to those who did not have lived experience. That made them important to each other—able to have the kind of compassion they needed to provide true peer support.

I welcome you to these pages, to explore what *Living Room* and raising mental health awareness was like starting in 2006. It's a piece of history that should not be forgotten.

Marja

CHAPTER ONE
Mental Health and the Church

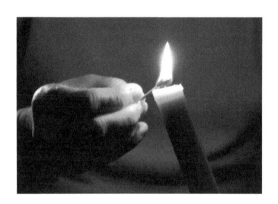

MENTAL HEALTH AND THE CHURCH IN 2006

As I start telling this story about *Living Room*, I want to remind readers of how mental health problems were regarded back in 2006. There was far less awareness than we have today. This was true In the secular world, but even more so in the church—the place where hurting individuals were hoping to find God's comfort and compassion.

There is nothing like a church family's support in keeping faith alive. Instead of receiving spiritual care, many who struggled were being hurt.

At the time *Living Room* was founded, troubled individuals were blamed for their problems. Instead of being comforted, they were made to feel ashamed.

Since 2012, the hard work of Sanctuary Mental Health Ministries has come along to make a difference. Before that time, I did all I could to better the lives of those who, like me, struggled with mental illness. I was passionate about it. It was the work God had given me to do, and I gave it my all.

I wrote articles and letters, presented at conferences, had speaking engagements, led a *Living Room* group, and planted more. I was also on the 100 Huntley Street Christian television show. Around the time of the first *Living Room* meeting, the Canadian Mental Health Association (CMHA), published an article, the writing of which, they had entrusted to me because I was able to write as a Christian. I copy the article here:

Church Support: the Good, the Bad and the Ugly
– September 2006

We all know how bad the stigma towards those with mental illness is in society. But I think stigma is at its worst when it presents itself in the church community. And, let's face it, there is a lot of ignorance, especially in that community. I think this is not only unfortunate, but also tragic.

All too often the message that comes from the pulpit is that we should be able to deal with all our emotional problems through spiritual means. Many Christians don't believe in the medical aspects of mental disorders and encourage their friends to "Stop taking those pills. Taking pills shows that you don't trust in God. If you're feeling down, you're probably not right with God. Confess your sins, and you'll be alright." Now this mistaken viewpoint is of course not present everywhere.

There are many of us, myself included, who find wonderful support in their churches. In fact I think the support from friends who share your faith is the best you can get. Those who try to emulate the character of Christ by sharing their non-judgmental, compassionate love with those who are suffering give better support than can be had in almost any other segment of society. They encourage their sick friends to follow their faith and to cling to the knowledge that God IS there, even if he doesn't seem to be. They become God's representatives to their hurting friend.

But bring into this picture a misunderstanding, uninformed church friend or pastor telling you that there's something wrong with your relationship with God, and the results could be tragic. In this kind of situation the church can do more damage than any other part of society.

When a person who is already feeling the pain and negativity of depression is told that the fault lies within himself or that he is possessed by a demon (yes, there are still some who believe this) – I can't imagine anything worse for a person with mental illness.

The biggest problem a newly diagnosed person has to overcome is the acceptance that she needs to take psychiatric medication. So many fight against treatment and thus have a huge struggle with recovery. The process of acceptance is difficult. How much worse it is for someone of faith to be told by their church friends not to take the medication – in fact, to be told the medication is somehow "evil". I recently read a pastor's blog claiming that the use of psychiatric medication was "sorcery."

Christians are called to be "followers of Christ." As such we need to love as he does. Our role is to be compassionate. It's God's role to judge, not ours. Dr. Harold G. Koenig, M.D., author of *New Light on Depression*, said that the unconditional love that Christ displayed and that Christians are called to emulate, is "the ultimate long-term antidote for depression." I believe that to be true.

It's through the love my church friends have shown me that I have come to fully grasp how deep God's love is. That helps me hang onto my faith, no matter what. This is what gives the courage and strength to continue, even when my road turns black.

Having faith is important to our mental well-being. We need people who share our faith to give us their unconditional love, as Christ does.

MY TESTIMONY, WRITTEN IN 2009

My Christian walk started in 1988 when I was going through a horrendous time with psychosis. I could see no other way to continue my life without God in it. I learned to lean on him to help me survive the symptoms of my illness. His deep love gave me the comfort I so often needed. Although my bipolar disorder was hard to live with, having Jesus in my life gave me joy. I wanted to follow him and to serve in the way I saw him serve.

I have lived with bipolar disorder as a person who didn't believe in God. And I've lived with bipolar illness as someone who learned to have faith in God. And, though my faith did not "heal" me, I have become a stronger person because of it.

Trusting in God has removed a lot of the fear I had. I don't become anxious as often. I know that I'm on a spiritual journey that will never end until I go to heaven. Some anxiety and some fear will always be part of my life. But I live with a hope that keeps me well more than I would otherwise be. And, though I know that depression will still periodically hit me - as it has quite a few times over the past 18 months—I've learned that every time I come back into the light, I'm a different person in some way. My moods teach me things, even if it's only to have better compassion for others who suffer in some way.

The Bible says "...*we rejoice in our sufferings, because we know that suffering produces perseverance; perseverance, character; and character, hope. And hope does not disappoint us, because God has poured out his love into our hearts by the Holy Spirit, who he has given us.*" (Romans 5:3-5)

Although suffering is painful, there *is* something about the pain that does build character.

But I think the greatest thing I've learned since I began following Christ, was that God loves me unconditionally, no matter what. When I go through the feelings of abandonment and darkness that come periodically, I try to remember Jesus who is well acquainted with those feelings. He also suffered greatly—all for us. God knows what our pain is like. When we suffer, he suffers with us. We are not alone. We can cling to this knowledge.

I have known of God's love for a long time, but I haven't always felt it, or grasped just how great it truly is. But when I did, I became more confident, more assured of my worth. And all I knew I wanted to do, was to work for him, to help others understand how wide and long and high and deep his love is.

Update from 2020: Life changes are bound to happen for all of us. I'm no exception. I had some unfortunate things happen to me that affected my illness in a big way. Things are quite different from what I've written above. But when I'm experiencing darkness or pain, I know that Jesus is always with me. Jesus understands my pain and helps me carry it.

CHAPTER TWO
Living Room is Born

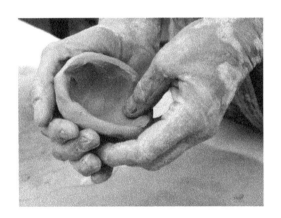

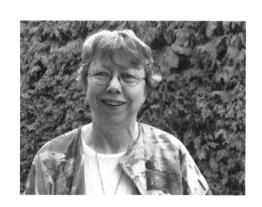

LIVING ROOM IS BORN

From early on I felt angry about the stigma attached to mental illness. I was angry at the injustice that caused individuals to feel shame about having an illness they couldn't help. It was unfair that they be looked down on, made to feel inferior to others. God called me to do all I could to better the situation. I have been devoting my life to this work.

The idea for a faith-based group came to me in early 2006 when I was attending a support group of the Mood Disorders Association of B.C. The group members had been going around the circle, telling what helps them cope best. When my turn came I was in a bit of a quandary. How would they feel if I told them God was more important than anything else to help me cope with my ups and downs? Would I embarrass them?

I did end up telling the group about my faith. After the meeting I was surprised to have two or three come and tell me about their own faith.

After the MDA meeting I realized groups were needed where mental health and faith could both be discussed together. At that time this wasn't possible anywhere. Not in the secular world, nor in the church. There needed to be a place where people who believe in God and needing support for their mental health, could gather.

I couldn't wait to put the plans for a faith-based mental health support group in motion. My pastor was supportive but cautious. I had to find a co-facilitator before I could do anything. Fortunately, one did come forward. The two of us did a lot of praying.

As I worked towards making Christian peer support a reality I frequently doubted myself. Who am I anyway to be doing something this big? I had never heard of faith-based groups addressing mental health problems. This was a brand new thing I was undertaking. Where do I start?

From 1993 I'd been fighting the stigma of mental illness, mostly addressing Christian audiences. Now I would be giving direct help to those with such illnesses. I would be giving spiritual care to people who had for too long been misunderstood—even ignored by the church. My work was expanding. No longer was I only speaking *about* them I was working *for* them.

The story of David and Goliath inspired me. I saw myself as the young David fighting the giant Philistine. I looked at Goliath as the immense problem of stigma. It was so huge and overwhelming that the head and feet could not be seen. Only the massive body. Where should I aim my attack? Where should I start? How could I possibly be strong enough or clever enough?

David's response when King Saul doubted his ability to fight Goliath encouraged me. *"Your servant has killed both the lion and the bear. This uncircumcised Philistine will be like one of them because he has defied the armies of the living God. The Lord who rescued me from the paw of the lion and the paw of the bear, will rescue me from the hand of this Philistine.* " (1 Samuel 17:36-37)

WHAT IS LIVING ROOM?

We called the group *Living Room*, a name coined by Dr. John Toews, a psychiatrist and author of *No Longer Alone: Mental Health and the Church*. Dr. Toews is a proponent of better church support for people with mental illness and helped inspire the organization of our group.

The founding *Living Room* became an outreach project in partnership with the Mood Disorders Association of BC (MDA), a secular organization that trained us how to facilitate.

We advertised in MDA's newsletter, as well as the local community newspapers. The calls trickled in at a steady pace until four months later we had twenty people on our list. Many others called as well, people who might join us in the future.

Though I focus on the participants, I mention my own struggles at group meetings. This tells them I am one of them.

When I talk about my feelings, others are encouraged to talk about theirs. We study scripture and share our suffering, always relieved to discover that others understand.

Relationships built on authentic sharing of our vulnerabilities become strong. Because we have all suffered, we have compassion for each other. We share a common language. When the participants believe in God and talk about how God works in their lives, the strength of our bond grows. Not only do we share similar emotional problems, but we also encourage each other's faith. We share God's love with each other.

What does *Living Room* offer? So many who live with mental health problems don't feel they belong anywhere. *Living Room* faith based support groups offer places where I don't think anyone feels out of place or on the outside looking in. Self-help groups like this offer good places to overcome feelings of alienation.

At *Living Room* each person is warmly welcomed. No matter what their emotional condition they are fully accepted. The open sharing of problems that are usually kept from people on the outside is healing. Because of this transparency, members come to love and appreciate each other for who they are. And with God at the centre and Jesus as our example how could it go wrong?

At one *Living Room* meeting earlier in the group's history, someone who was having a rough time shared that she had no

Christian support at all until she started coming to *Living Room*. Churches she attended had not been open to hearing about such problems. The pastor of the church she currently attended knew of her illness but warned her not to let anyone in the congregation know about it. They wouldn't understand.

As a result, she had no Christian friends with whom she could be open about her struggles. She spent three weeks in hospital not feeling she could tell anyone. No one from her church prayed for her or visited this lady. This is only one of many individuals with mental health issues who are starving for the spiritual support often lacking in churches.

Living Room groups fill that hole because they are facilitated by individuals who have mental health challenges themselves. They are best equipped to understand the issues members deal with and they are best able to have compassion for the people they lead. When group leaders show their vulnerability, briefly telling about their own struggles and how God works in their life, others are encouraged to open up. This kind of facilitation is the key to a good group. Churches need people like these to work with the pastor in organizing such a group.

ANNOUNCING LIVING ROOM AT CHURCH
– September 2006

The pastor invited me to talk to the congregation about the support group. To tell them why I had decided to form the group. This would lead into his sermon on building authentic community.

When my time came to speak, the pastor introduced the *"Living Room"* as the name we are giving the group. I started by telling everyone that I had lived with bipolar disorder for forty years and that I cope by taking medications, trusting in God, and through the support of good friends. I told them that I'm not always as good as this. I often struggle.

I quoted the beginning of 2 Corinthians: that *"God, the Father of compassion and the God of all comfort...comforts us in all our troubles, so that we can comfort those in any trouble with the comfort we ourselves have received from God."* "One good thing about having a lot of troubles like I've had," I said, "is that I've received a *lot* of compassion from God. It's helped me realize how real he is."

Then I told them about the countless people who have depression, anxiety and bipolar disorders, how most of them are alone with their troubles, ashamed to share them with others. I told them how wrong I thought that was. Not only do they suffer from the symptoms of their disorder, but they are also made to feel ashamed. They should not have to suffer alone. They need to realize that there are others who share such troubles. There needs to be a place where they can openly share what's in their hearts.

I told them about the secular support groups where people don't feel comfortable talking about God. And I told them how, at the church's Bible studies, people are often uncomfortable talking about their mental health issues. *Living Room* will be a place where they can talk freely about their faith *and* their mental health issues.

The purpose of *Living Room* is for members to provide each other with love and support; to remind each other how great God's love is; and to seek transformation in their lives.

I found it interesting to see which people talked to me afterwards and which looked at me, seemingly not knowing what to say. But one couple came up to me and very much wanted to join. They told me I was courageous.

When I began writing about my struggles with bipolar, I knew I would be giving up a lot. With the publication of *Riding the Roller Coaster* my life became, literally, an open book. It continues to be that. I guess it was a form of sacrifice. But I feel steely strong inside, wanting more than ever, to bust that ugly stigma that causes so much grief. So what if there are some people that think I'm odd? They don't know me. I have absolutely nothing to be ashamed of. I have many friends and feel loved and that's all I need. God gave me a purpose and this is what I'll continue giving my life to.

PREPARATIONS

We were surprised at how well the small announcements in the papers were noticed. The calls started coming in. "What do you mean by "faith based" mental health support?" I think some thought it was too good to be true. Many wanted to talk, Christians who had been hurt at church.

The people who came to *Living Room* were hurting, not only from the symptoms of their mental illness, but more so from the way they had been treated. Here they were welcomed to a spiritual home that accepted them and their mental health difficulties. Their faith and mental health were addressed together. *Living Room* became their church.

Living Room, and the light it gradually brought to Christian understanding was much needed. The message of Jesus Christ and his care for the outcast brought comfort and emotional strength to individuals who had been hungry for spiritual care.

HOW AND WHERE DID WE MEET?

The founding group, facilitated by myself and co-facilitated by Janice K met at Brentwood Park Alliance Church in Burnaby two afternoons a month with lunch provided. A second group started a month later, meeting two evenings a month at New Life Community Church in Burnaby. It was facilitated by Mark J and co- facilitated by Graeme H.

At Brentwood church we met in a large, cavernous hall in the basement—not the most cozy meeting place. What helped was putting a table in the centre of the hall covered with a colourful tablecloth. A centerpiece was in the middle, and for a few years we provided dishes of chocolates. Boxes of Kleenex completed the setting.

As the group grew, the table grew. We put several long tables together until it became huge. Gathering around one single table was a must for me. It spelled togetherness. Easier to talk with each other and more comfortable for having lunch and coffee.

My group was an outreach ministry, drawing people from the community. They came from far and wide. Members came as they felt the need, so we never knew how many would come. It was always a surprise. Almost always, one or two new people came. Many came by word of mouth. The day before the meeting, we always called to encourage everyone to come. It helped them feel connected.

The introductions were conducted much like AA. Going around the table, each person gave their first name and—if they wished—what their diagnosis is. Doing so helps them feel there's nothing to be ashamed of. After prayer we went into devotion time. It's an interactive devotional where the facilitator introduced a theme and everyone is given a chance to have input.

Before going into sharing groups, we prayed, asking God to fill us with his love and to help us share that love with each other. I believe that prayer had an impact on the way the sharing time went. There was a lot of love in the group.

Living Room is important to the people who come. Some of them have been hurt by misunderstanding friends. All of us at *Living Room*, including the leaders, understand what it's like to live with mood disorders. And so, we know how to support each other. By sharing our stories we find out we're not alone.

THE FIRST MEETING

On Friday September 15, 2006 I wrote this in my blog:

Today was the big day. We had our first meeting of the support group. It was a tiny group; there were only four of us: me, my co-facilitator and two others.

A few weeks ago I was nervous about facilitating. But today I felt prepared, eager to begin. I felt comfortable in the role. I can sense that this is work God genuinely wants me to do.

Fifteen minutes into the meeting, almost having given up on anyone else coming, we heard the heavy footsteps of a man clumping down the long staircase. When he appeared he surprised us. He looked somewhat dishevelled and, to be honest, he scared me a bit. After introductions, we started discussing the day's topic, *Fear*. After a long interval the man surprised us with his gruff voice. "I have fear." This began our first sharing time. Terry was a person I cared a lot about. He stayed with us for many years, sharing his fears, but also sharing his love for God.

I know the group will only grow gradually. It takes courage to join something new like this, especially if you're not well. But even if there were only a handful of us, it would be worthwhile. I think all of us who were there at that first tiny meeting got something out of that first meeting.

Soon I will be getting back to work on my book, *A Firm Place to Stand*. I know that one thing I will have to write about, is this program. I want to describe how we run it and the benefits it provides, not only to people in our church but to the community. Perhaps readers will be inspired to start such a group in their own church.

Today I'm thankful for all the friends who are supporting me and my work. I know there are people praying for me and I can sense it helping. Today I very much felt God's presence.

LIVING ROOM TESTIMONIES

- "I encouraged my friend to google bipolar to find out more. I think the desire to dispel the stigma of our disease is rubbing off on me. In my small way I'm trying to educate others that I come across and it's amazing how when you share your vulnerabilities people often open up about themselves and about the people that are close to them that suffer from mental illness."

• "I'm frequently encouraged to hear how important *Living Room* is when I hear the stories from members of the group. At one meeting a man his wife, strong members of their church, never felt free to talk about his bipolar disorder there. They kept his disease a dark secret, a burden for which they received no spiritual support. Being able to talk about his problems in the Christian setting we provided gave him tremendous relief. People like this need to have the freedom to share their mental health problems with their church family."

• "After a sermon I heard at church over 10 years ago I felt God nudging me to start an evening group at my church. I was not feeling like a leader but felt called to step out of my comfort zone. Having an evening group would be available to people working during the day and also there wasn't a west side group. I had really enjoyed going to the group in Burnaby and it helped me understand my new bipolar diagnosis. Plus when my dad ended his life by suicide in 2007 the members there were very supportive. I've been told many times from members of my group that *Living Room* is important to them. This is the only place that they can be honest and authentic about how they are feeling, their struggles and frustrations. They know that everyone understands. The important aspect of being prayed for was really the difference that others groups did not have."

• A comment from early Living Room history: "When I told my friend about my support group for mood disorders and what a blessing it was, she asked 'isn't it depressing to be around a bunch of "crazy" people?' I said, 'No way, it's a safe place to support each other in our common brokenness and to realize you're not the only one to feel this way. In that setting, I've learned that it's an invisible disease but not any different than diabetes and to dispel the stigma and shame associated with mental illness. I'm learning that my condition is not a curse but could be a blessing. In my lows I get a sense of the emotional pain people can go through. "

• Living room group is one of the only safe places where I feel I can be completely myself. I don't feel ashamed to share that I am medicated, that I struggle with suicidal thoughts or that I have hallucinations. It's an understanding community where I don't have to put on a brave face and pretend I have it all together. I can pray and talk about the most vulnerable experiences of living with bipolar disorder with people who are empathetic because they have similar issues. I'm a leader at the Tenth Church group. I treasure the times to connect with this group and always leave feeling uplifted. I feel seen, heard and loved.

CHAPTER THREE
Spreading the Word

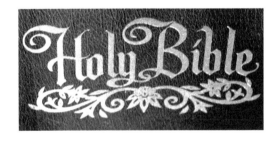

SPREADING THE WORD

The first two years of *Living Room* were busy ones. I was consumed with a passion to get the word out. Not only about *Living Room*, but also about bringing mental health awareness to churches. I wanted to help them understand that they, with their knowledge of Christ's love, are in the best position to help people with mental health issues.

SERMON PROPOSAL

On November 27, 2006, just over a month since the beginning of *Living Room*, I sent out this sermon proposal to as many church leaders as I could think of. I was heavily into blogging and asked my blogging pals to pass it on. The National Association for Mental Illness (NAMI) ran it for a long time on their Faithnet website.

Dear Friends,
A friend of mine, someone with bipolar disorder, recently said to me, "*I've gone to church nearly all my life and I've just heard about mental illnesses mentioned once, and just in passing. When I was hospitalized, some people came from the church, but they just prayed for the devil to leave me.*"

As someone who also lives with bipolar disorder, a medical illness, I find this tragic. It's painful for a person who is already suffering to be told she's not right with

God. It damages a person's relationship with her Christian friends and her church. Some even come to believe that it *is* the devil that is the cause of their troubles and refuse to take the medication that would help them survive.

Would a person in hospital because of a heart attack, a stroke, or Alzheimer's be prayed for in this way? Can you imagine how that could make a person feel?

I believe churches should, at least once a year, receive a message from the pulpit on the truths about mental illness. I know that pastors don't usually preach about illnesses, but in this case, congregants need to learn how to separate the spiritual from the medical. Too many are uninformed and make things worse because they don't know how to best support people who are going through emotional trauma. The kind of support such individuals need is similar to the support people with physical illness need. Practical help with things like meals and transportation. A sympathetic ear. Church leaders can help their church family learn how to provide this.

There are two excellent opportunities each year for such a sermon. This upcoming year, May 7 - 13 is Mental Health Week. In October there is a Mental Health Awareness Week as well.

Here is a link to an article I recently wrote which will give some ideas on what good church support looks like.

https://www.heretohelp.bc.ca/visions/stigma-and-discrimination-vol2/mental-disorders-the-result-of-sin (2005)

If you know someone who is a pastor, could you please forward this message on to him or her? You would be doing a big service for the many who suffer from mental illness and need to be understood.

VANCOUVER SUN ARTICLE

In February 2007, at the request of the BC Mood Disorders Association of BC (MDA), I was asked to do an interview with a journalist from The Vancouver Sun. The paper was doing a three-part weekend report on depression. It was an excellent series and I was happy to see them doing such a thorough job of it. Big front-page attention plus a two-page spread inside each paper.

A photographer came and photographed me holding my book, *Riding the Roller Coaster*. And where did he photograph me? At the base of the roller coaster in Vancouver. He took many shots, far more than I thought he would need.

But the next day I learned why when I opened the Saturday paper. My photo could not be missed. It was prominently displayed on the front cover. Such a surprise.

A DIZZY SOUL

In June 2007 I wrote the following:

I'll be going to Bible study in a little while and I know that one question our facilitator, Mary, told us she will be asking is, "How is your soul?" I would have to answer that it's rather dizzy right now, though it is improving. I'm beginning to settle down. Better able to focus on the jobs at hand.

For such a long time my main goal has been to reduce the stigma in the church toward those with mental health problems. For so long I'd been striving to educate Christians by writing articles, promoting a pastor's mental health workshop and writing a book. But now things are coming together.

Canadianchristianity.com has asked me to contribute regular articles on the topic of mental health and the church. The more I think about it, the more I realize this is a wonderful opportunity. This is exactly where I need to be. God is good.

In May their website published my testimony. Soon they will be publishing an article I wrote a couple of years ago for the Canadian Mental Health Association (CMHA), *Mental Illness: The Result of Sin*?

Other questions we will have to be prepared to answer this morning is, "How have you seen God at work in and through your life since we last met?" and "What God-given dream are you nurturing?" My answers to these will be easy. God has been at work leading me to fulfill my dream and, bit by bit, it's becoming a reality.

That isn't all. Another great thing is happening. A woman in Abbotsford, a town forty-five minutes from here, is working to start a *Living Room* group in her church. This could be the beginning of my vision to see *Living Room* groups in many churches.

Not long ago, a call came from a therapist wanting to learn about *Living Room*. He is hoping to send his Christian clients to us. So often they feel they're bad Christians when they're depressed. They don't want to take medication. *Living Room* would be helpful because it draws from the Bible and recognizes the medical nature of mood disorders. It's amazing where God leads us when we let him!

When we do the work God wants us to do with a positive and prayerful spirit, things do come together. And what a joy it is to see that happen!

LIVING ROOM MANUALS

After a successful Mental Health service at my church in May 2007 I realized the formation of more groups was needed and decided to go to work to help that happen. The demand was greater than my church and I could adequately respond to. I decided to write a manual as a tool for churches who wished to do what we had done. But to do a proper job we needed to get some funding from an organization that shared our vision. I didn't wait. I began writing.

In August that year, a two-part set of *Living Room* manuals was ready for printing. One described how to set up a group. The other described how to facilitate. We were wondering how to fund the printing but ended up with support we hadn't expected.

The Mennonite Supportive Care Society (MCCSC) (now Communitas), a ministry which supports people with disabilities, sent a large number of copies to pastors, with a letter promoting the *Living Room* concept. Their purchase helped pay for some of the printing.

Dr. Phillip Long, my psychiatrist, was a big supporter. He always told me how Alcoholics Anonymous had also started as a Christian ministry and grew to be more than had ever been expected. He believed that *Living Room* could evolve in the same way.

When he saw one of the manuals and how it was presented in a report cover he asked, "Is that all it is? How much is it going to cost to publish this properly?" When I told him, he immediately pulled out his cheque book and wrote a cheque.

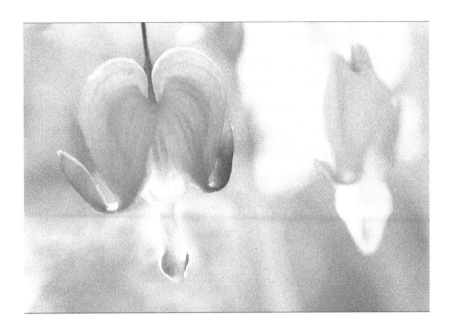

Living Room

mood disorders support group
facilitator's guide

artnership with

DISORDERS ASSOCIATION
BRITISH COLUMBIA

*"Be shepherds of God's flock
that is under your care..."*
I Peter 5:2

NEW MANUAL READY, AUGUST 24, 2007

In a joyous notice on my blog, I wrote the following on August 24, 2007:

After a lot of work, checking and re-checking, having them checked by others, having them professionally edited and then beautifully printed, the two manuals are finally finished. They're sitting in open boxes in our hallway where I can look at them as I pass and feel good about it all. I've received a lot of interest from people who want to have copies. How gratifying! And when I think of how much good this could end up doing...!

Living Room is a Christian self-help group for people with depression, anxiety and bipolar disorders. Ideally facilitators should have one of these problems. They will be better able to identify—better able to support. The group is in partnership with a mood disorder association. This helps avoid the danger of trying to spiritualize the problems too much - something Christian groups need to watch out for.

I want to share with you a bit about *Living Room*—some of the things I cover in my new manual.

Neat thing is: "You get help, you give help, and—in the process—help yourself."

It's obvious how participants can benefit from this place where they can share their troubles with others, at the same time discussing their faith. Finding out they're not alone helps them gather encouragement and strength.

But how does the church benefit?

1. The church responds to Christ's call to love and help people in need.
2. It helps people who are often shunned in the community.
3. It helps break down the stigma of mental illness by promoting prayer and support for the participants.
4. It helps make mental illness an acceptable topic of conversation, encouraging others to be open about their struggles and search out treatment and support.
5. It gives members of the congregation opportunities to gain a better understanding about mental health issues.

I'm frequently encouraged to hear how important *Living Room* is when I hear the stories from members of the group. At the last meeting there was a man his wife who were strong members of his church but never felt free to talk about his bipolar disorder there. They kept his disease a dark secret—a burden for which they received no spiritual support. Being able to talk about his problems in the Christian setting we provided gave him a tremendous relief. It was a release he very much needed.

There are many stories—too many to share here. But I feel a passion for this program and think it needs to extend to communities everywhere. Yet I know it will take time. People have to feel free to share their problems with the disorder with their church family.

Once again, I offer this manual to you. Even if you're not ready to start up, I believe it will be an inspiration that will help you see what is possible when there is a place where people can freely talk about their mental health difficulties in the light of their faith.

I promised to let you know the cost of these books (though they're only 20 and 24 pages, they're more than just booklets).

- Creating Living Room helps people with mood disorders and church leaders learn the Living Room concept and how to set up a group. Cost: $2.50
- Facilitating Living Room gives facilitators guidance and encouragement. Cost: $3.25.
- Cost of postage and handling for one book or the two together is the same. Within Canada: $2.50. To the US: $4.00. That's under $10 for the two. We're only covering our costs.

(Authors' Note: These are no longer available.)

100 HUNTLEY STREET INTERVIEW

I was excited in October 2007, but worried too. The national Christian TV show, 100 Huntley Street had approached me about doing an interview. They wanted to hear about my life and ministry. The reporter found me through articles I had published on canadianchristianity.com.

This was a dream come true. I had wanted to be on that show for a long time. Such an excellent venue to talk about faith and mental illness. I had planned to approach them once my book, *A Firm Place to Stand*, had come out. It was amazing that they had now approached me instead.

The reporter/producer spent an entire day with me, interviewing me, taping a session of *Living Room*, and interviewing my pastor and a couple of members of the group.

The reason I'm a bit worried is because in recent days, when talking about *Living Room*, I've found it hard to express myself. A lot of fumble mouth.

Perhaps I've been steeped in too much mental health work lately. My son and his wife are creating a *Living Room* website, a job that requires a lot of input from me. A new *Living Room* has started in Abbotsford and another is trying to start up in that same city. I've been working on devotional samples to share with other groups as well. I also get phone calls from people needing support. And then there was the book proposal I sent to an agency recently.

There are other things in life that I seem to have little time for. I must do some work around the house. Start trying to cook some decent meals again. Balance my life.

Yes, I must come down to earth again.

A FIRM PLACE TO STAND LAUNCHED JULY 19, 2008

What do you do when you're so happy that, waking up at 3:30 in the morning, you can't get back to sleep again? This happened Sunday morning. I was too happy to sleep. I felt like there was something I should do with such happiness. Dance or something. But I mostly just sat around...feeling that flood of good feelings—not able to do a thing with it.

The reason for this great joy was the launch party on Saturday. It turned out beautifully. The weather was beautiful, the food was great, the garden was full of flowers, and everyone was happy.

Seventy of my friends and acquaintances had gathered in our yard to celebrate the launch of my new book, *A Firm Place to Stand*. I had started writing this book around the time I founded *Living Room*. The purpose was to help readers realize that it's possible to be a good Christian and have a mental illness too.

Some of the guests were people who I had supported through hard times. It was wonderful to have them here for this occasion. Good to see them doing better. People from my church came, from my writer's group, from *Living Room*, family members, neighbors, and old friends. A couple of people from the Mood Disorders Association of BC came as well.

I was fortunate to have friends helping me with this big event. My daughter-in-law Jeannette, a cook who loves to experiment, made some interesting appetizers, including dates stuffed with goat cheese. My friend Shelley made a variety of hot appetizers and sold books for me. And I don't know what I would have done without my friend Mary. She made sure the food tables were always well stocked and was on her feet through the entire event. Shelley's and Mary's husbands and my husband worked hard the day before putting up seven canopies. What a lot of support I received!

A few days before, as soon as I had received a copy of the book I took it to my 94 year old mother. I got such a huge kick showing it to her, watching as she read what I had written about her. Her eyesight is failing, yet the typesetting is clear and easy to read, so she had no trouble with it. I'll always remember how her eyes traveled across the page, her face intent. I should have taken a picture.

Now—in the words of my friend Mary—a new chapter of my life will begin. I will need to promote the book, using it to encourage Christians who have mental illness and to get the word out about the importance of faith-based support. It's time to get to work trying to make a further dent in the stigma that exists. My focus the Christian church.

GARDEN PARTY

I wrote *A Firm Place to Stand* to show that having a mental illness does not mean you're not a good Christian.

The garden party was a wonderful setting for the launch. Colourful. Fun. A great mix of friends and acquaintances. Children painting a mural. My friend Janice face painting. Delicious food.

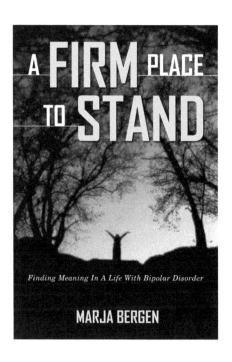

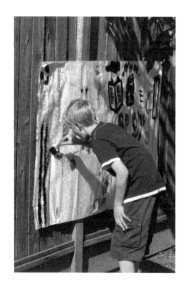

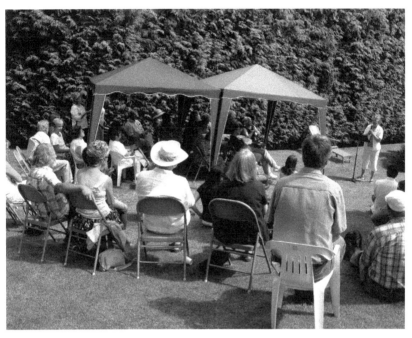

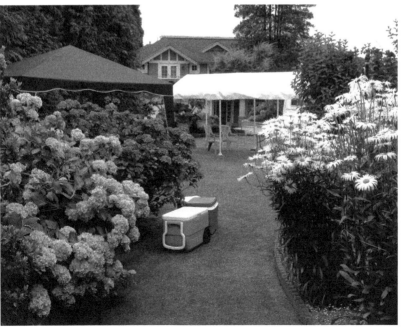

OVERWHELMED

In August 2008 I wrote the following:

I'm healthy but—I think quite understandably—overwhelmed with all I have on my plate. I feel as though I'm trying to live the lives of half a dozen people, all at one time. And I don't know how I'm going to manage all I need to do. In fact, I don't think I will manage. I'll have to decide on what is most important and be efficient with my time. Good thing I've just had a holiday and I do have energy. I only wish there were more of me.

I've been studying how to publicize and market books...and wow, all the things I should be doing! No wonder publicists are so costly. They have a huge job. And not being able to afford one, I will have to do that myself. I need to do this as well as I can, because I believe *A Firm Place to Stand* is a book that will help fight stigma, and that's an important cause. I want the book to be read by many.

The Vancouver Sun had a series about mental illness last week, pointing out the effects of stigma on the welfare of people with mental illness. It's a terrible situation that needs to change. I believe my book and the things I have to say can be a building block in promoting such change. I want to speak to the media. I want people to learn more. I want to help compassion grow.

But I also have a 94-year-old mom who needs me. And I have *Living Room* and its people. Not just my group, but the other groups I'd like to help grow. I want to leave time for the people who come to me for support. I want to write articles. I want to blog.

This will be a busy week. I'm getting ready for a family barbecue at our house. We will be going through some of my mother-in-law's things to divide up the memories of her between us. I still need to go through her huge mess of boxes and organize what's inside. I'll need to clean the house and cook.

I'm overwhelmed!

Today I'm in a position to build mental health awareness in the church. To show how they can support people with mental illness. I feel the responsibility in a big way. But how can I best do it with the few resources of time I have? Where should I concentrate my efforts?

Please, God, lead me in the best way to go. I know I'm not on my own with this. This is, after all, your work and not my own. I shouldn't worry so much. I should realize that the burden is not all mine to carry. Help me to take aim with my writing tools and publicity in a way that will do the most good.

LIVING ROOM BECOMES A BURDEN

In June 2009 I wrote the following: Things haven't been good. Every once in a while a good day and every once in a while an absolutely horrendous day.

I am grateful for the good weather we've had. I've been able to spend the early morning hours sitting on the patio, listening to the birds, enjoying the flowers, aware of God's presence. Those times have been healing.

One of my worst problems lately has been Living Room. This ministry that always gave me such joy has become a burden. I feel alone with the responsibility—and it is a big responsibility. Is it the depression that is making it feel like a burden? Or is the burden causing the depression? I'm not sure which it is.

My own group isn't a problem. I have lots of help there. It's the bigger picture of Living Room: raising awareness within the church, helping churches learn how to support people with mental illness. That's where I must have support.

I need a lot of prayer right now for someone to come alongside to share in the work. I need someone who will share this vision with me. Depressed and unable to do more than absolute essentials, I complained to my church and asked for prayer to help someone materialize.

Every once in a while my mood dips dangerously low. And yet I must trust God. I must remember that he is in charge. And I must remember to keep talking to him, aware of his presence, grateful for his love and his goodness. I'm trying to hang onto God as well as I can.

Although I have asked my church repeatedly for help, no one has come forward.

My counselor, my husband and friends have tried to tell me not to think so much about always doing for other people. They believed I should *"dwell in the land and enjoy safe pasture."* (Psalm 37:3) "Relax," they say. But I couldn't agree with them.

Psalm 37 also says to *"Trust in the Lord and DO GOOD"*. I can't simply "dwell in the land" when there are things wrong with it. I'm not able to rest knowing there are people with mental health issues who are made to feel they are less than others. How can I possibly relax when I see such injustice? Aren't we called to follow Christ's example of love and acceptance?

As I look back on this in 2020, I have spent twenty-six years trying to make the world a better place for those living with mental health problems. That's God's clear call on my life. I don't think I could ever stop.

Matthew 5:6 speaks powerfully to me: *Blessed are those who hunger and thirst for righteousness, for they will be filled.*

LIVING ROOM AT MENTAL HEALTH CONFERENCE

November 2009: My moods continue to go up and down. And when I feel ok, it's as though I'm walking a tightrope, trying to maintain my balance so I don't fall one way or another.

Amazing how many symptoms there are to watch out for. And each time one of those symptoms shows itself, I have to put a different coping mechanism into place. Read a different psalm, pray a different prayer.

There are the lonely feelings, the poor eating, overwhelmed feelings where I can't see how I can possibly manage doing the many things I need to do, unable to organize a list. Little things seem like big things. I've even had moments thinking I couldn't go on. Thank God those moments have been brief ones.

I will have to walk my tightrope well. Do all the right things. Stay well.

I'm preparing for *Living Room* on Friday. Also preparing for the *Into the Light: Transforming Mental Health in Canada Conference* coming up November 27th. This is a national conference put on by the *Mental Health Commission of Canada*, Vancouver Coastal Health, and Simon Fraser University.

PRESENTATION POSTER

Faith-based support for people with
mood disorders, including depression,
anxiety, and bipolar disorders

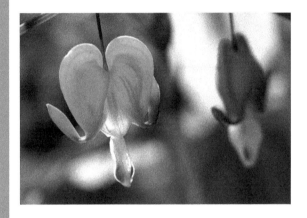

Reducing
stigma in
the church

OUR MISSION

Living Room is a network of Christian peer-facilitated support groups for people with mood disorders, creating places of safety, acceptance, understanding, healing and community. Support groups arc sponsored by local churches and para-church agencies in partnership with mental health profes-sionals, agencies and associations.

Manuals can be downloaded
free of charge:
www.livingroomsupport.org

Contact: Marja Bergen
marja@livingroomsupport.org

"We get help, give help, and help ourselves."

FAITH

BENEFITS for Living Room Participants

"...to grasp how wide and long and high and deep is the love of Christ"
Ephesians 3:18

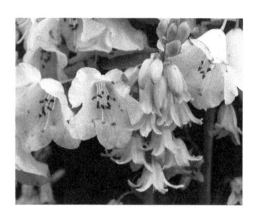

A SAFE PLACE TO COME and:

- Not be alone,
- Find understanding, encouragement, and acceptance,
- Share your struggles openly in confidence,
- Meditate on the Scriptures and through prayer,
- Receive healing by sharing with people who understand,
- Overcome feelings of guilt and shame,
- See the stigma of mental illness vanish through sharing with fellow sufferers.

"I am a Christian, but I feel so very alone in my battles and struggles. I know I shouldn't, but I feel ashamed and embarrassed to ask for prayer related to my disorder. I need His strength, but I also yearn for the support of those who hold the same worldview/belief system."

Living Room will have a presentation there. I'll have an opportunity to interact with conference attendees and tell them about it. This is exciting because it will be our first opportunity at a mainstream national conference to showcase what we do. An opportunity to highlight the importance of faith to mental well-being. To show what churches have it in their power to do, if they only would.

To tell the truth, at the event I felt rather small, on my own representing *Living Room*. On my own promoting a faith approach to mental health issues at such a major conference. I was grateful to Vicki Rogers from the BC Mood Disorders Association (MDA) who came to stand with me when my turn came to interact with attendees.

I went to several presentations and took opportunities to speak up for faith-based support when discussions allowed it. At an evening Wine and Cheese event, someone from Simon Fraser University's Coop Radio introduced himself. He was curious about how church and mental health could mix. After talking for awhile, he ended up taping an interview which was later broadcast.

What an exciting time that was! By the time the conference ended, I didn't feel so small anymore. Just extremely glad to have had the opportunity.

EIRANA SUPPORT

In April 2011, I gave a speech for the Reformed Church's Eirana Support Service's organization. It was well attended. The audience was eager to hear what I had to say. It felt good to speak, without any nervousness. The topics I covered:

- Finding meaning as a person with mental illness
- What can we do about the stigma?
- How can the church help?
- Christian peer support – *Living Room*
- Hope for future *Living Room* groups

Afterwards, a man who struggled with depression came to talk to me. He told me how he would like to be part of a Living Room group but did not feel he could facilitate. But he also told me how he was sitting on a park bench awhile back when a person—out of the blue—told him her life story and her struggles. He told me how good it made him feel. Without knowing it, he was doing Living Room work. In my estimation, he's a person who could facilitate.

Yet I know how scary it can feel. I was scared as well before I started my group the first time.

But I came to think of what it truly is. It's not my work at all. It's God's work. All I have to do is to be his feet and hands and voice. All the power comes from him who gives us strength. We only need to follow him.

HOW THINGS ARE CHANGING!

In June 2011 I had a meeting with Dr. Sharon Smith and Caroline Penhale who founded Sanctuary Mental Health Ministries. They are presenting workshops to give church congregations the tools they need to help those amongst them who live with mental illness. Living Room is partnering with this new organization.

This is exciting. These two professionals can broach the problem of stigma in a way I'm not able. And I fight stigma in a different way than they can. We come at the problem from two different perspectives and balance each other out. It's a great arrangement. We're gradually learning how we can best work together.

On September 17th Sharon and Caroline will speak at a workshop we're having to introduce churches to the Living Room concept. We hope this will lead to new groups for the Vancouver area.

I remember a time not too many years ago, before I wrote A Firm Place to Stand and before Living Room, when I tried to interest various seminaries in town in having someone speak to their counselling students about mental illness. Nothing happened. There was no interest. Maybe I just didn't have the credentials. I guess I wasn't someone who could have her thoughts seriously considered.

But things are changing. On November 9th Sharon Smith will be presenting a three-hour lecture at Regent College in Vancouver on mental health recovery in the church. Caroline Penhale and I will be speaking as well. I will tell my story and talk about the Living Room support ministry.

Faith communities are increasingly starting to see that they have a role to play when one of their congregants struggles with mental illness. And the medical community is starting to recognize that a person's faith plays a big part in his physical and emotional well-being. Sharon and Sanctuary is playing a big role in creating better understanding in both worlds.

The talk at Regent went well. I felt calm—exceedingly so. Not nervous, not shaking as I had been the days before the talks. I knew that friends were praying for me. Trouble was— and I feel bad about this—I'm pretty sure I talked far longer than I should have. Sharon ran out of time at the end and had to cram an hour of material into half an hour. I felt bad about that.

My talk about Living Room at the end of the lecture went much better. I was able to fit everything into five minutes, yet I felt I had said all that was needed. The note I ended on was that it would be wonderful if the whole church could be like Living Room. A place where people can be authentic and not have to hide the painful things they live with because of shame.

A LONG DISTANCE RACE

In December 2011 I wrote the following:

Much has changed since 2006 when I started the *Living Room* ministry. This ministry is now reaching far and wide. Currently there are sixteen groups, and more are forming. I'm grateful for how far God has taken it.

I've been wondering though, how long I can keep leading it. I've been having a lot of troubles. Loss of memory, disorganization, having normal or high moods followed quickly by depression, often with suicidal ideation.

And I wonder, is this the way it's always going to be for me? Is this a permanent condition caused by old age setting in? That is indeed a worry. I have to consider what needs to be done.

How I would love to find someone to take my place! Someone who I could at least prepare to take over leadership from me.

My pastor recently very wisely pointed me to Hebrews 11 and 12. He showed how with *Living Room* I blazed a trail like the biblical figures described. What a great privilege that has been! But I might not realize my goal. I never actually expect to destroy stigma. All I can hope for is to reduce it.

Yet I did hope and pray to have *Living Room* groups in churches readily available to as many people as possible. I hoped to start a movement towards reaching that goal. That was my prayer, whether voiced or not.

My prayer is that this *will* indeed be a movement that will catch fire. I pray that the *Living Room* candle that God helped me light will become a blaze of enlightenment in churches everywhere. I pray that all Christians living with mental illness will find themselves able to comfortably talk about their troubles. I pray that they will be able to truly be themselves, authentic members of their church families who can be open about who they are and what they deal with.

I pray for empathy and sympathy. For the elimination of feelings of shame. I pray that the church will be a source of comfort for people dealing with emotional difficulties. And, if the source of the problem is medical, I pray that it will be recognized as such and that the church could somehow work with medical staff to see that needs are met. I also pray that medical staff will work alongside the church where spiritual help is needed.

Erasing stigma is a long-distance race, one I will personally not give up fighting as long as I am able. I'm sure I will not see the finish line in my lifetime. But I have faith that—with God's help—a better life for Christians with mental illness will be possible. In the way God has helped me, God will help others carry the cause to the finish line.

SEEKING UNDERSTANDING

In January 2012, my devotional planner quoted Job 17:11: *"My days have passed, my plans are shattered, and so are the desires of my heart."*

The thoughts below the quote say, so correctly: "Plans give you energy and keep you moving forward. When plans get shattered so does your heart. The Lord can renew your plans or give you new plans. And when that happens your heart will be restored."

Job's old life with his plans were shattered. How I understand his feelings, though my situation isn't nearly as bad. I grieve the loss of my ability to function in a dependable way. And I do feel in great need of a new project —something without stress, something creative, something that will give me purpose, a God-given purpose. I believe if I had a good project to focus on, I would recover much sooner.

Living Room isn't shattered. It can't be. There will, I trust, be more capable individuals to carry it on. It's a movement. Manuals and other supportive materials are all available free of charge on the website. All we need is someone who will answer emails asking for info and someone who will supply encouragement where needed.

I just pray that I'll recover and that God will help me get stronger.

Any time I've had mental health problems I've turned to a creative project to restore my heart and give me a sense of excitement about life again. This is what I'm exploring now. I would like to create some kind of devotional book, including photographs. How I would love a project like that!! This is the idea I'm developing now.

I long to have my illness understood!

What do friends think of me? What do they think of my frequent ups and downs? I worry that they are allowing those moods to colour what they consider my personality to be. But my moods are not me. I can't help my moods.

I'm down so much. Yet I'm a positive thinker with big goals to reduce the stigma of mental illness. On behalf of the many who suffer as I do, I try to help others understand what it means to live with bipolar disorder so that they'll be more compassionate.

And yet, even people close to me misunderstand and withhold the support I need.

However, a friend pointed out to me that these people probably have enough problems of their own. Sometimes they just can't handle another thing. That's something I need to take into account. My fear though is that my moods make them think ill of me.

Who can I go to in times of deep darkness when I can't see my way clear, when I want to die and I just need someone to talk to and pray with?

My husband is a wonderful supporter. A patient man who has made a good life possible for me. But he doesn't have faith in God like I do. If he did, things would be so much different. I wouldn't need to depend as much on other friends.

God is number one in my life. I value my relationship with him. But when dark moods come I need a friend to remind me of his love and trustworthiness. A spiritual weakness of mine? Perhaps. But I know it's a common problem for people with depression.

MISSIONS FEST

In January 2012, *Living Room* had a booth at Missions Fest — a stressful but exciting affair. Caroline Penhale and Sharon Smith from Sanctuary, joined us in our booth. Walking around the exhibition hall, we appeared to be the only presenter there with a focus on mental health. I was glad to be there to help bring awareness to faith-based mental health needs.

In 2013 *Living Room* again had a booth. Many people stopped by to get information. People with mood disorders, people who had friends or family members with mood disorders. Others were simply happy to see that someone representing the church was addressing the problem of mental illness.

We had a couple of extra chairs in front of the booth for people who wanted to sit and talk. Some told stories of how the church had totally misunderstood the medical nature of mood disorders and prayed over unconfessed sins in an effort to heal the person. We talked about the pain this causes. We talked about the stigma in the church. We talked about their personal needs.

One woman walking by our booth exclaimed, "It's about time!"

MONDAY MORNING REFLECTIONS

In February 2013 I began the publication of *Reflections on Scripture*, devotions that were sent out via email to everyone who had approached me for support since *Living Room* started. At the time of this writing in 2020 there are 230 on the list.

The Reflections are designed specifically for people with mental health issues who don't have access to a *Living Room* group. The writings provide encouragement and support. From the beginning, the response was good. It's clear that people are being helped.

These writings have been important. Not only do they benefit the reader, but they help me a great deal as well. Writing those devotionals brings me close to God as I search for the message he wants to pass on.

Writing anchors me when I have trouble with my stability or when I'm struggling emotionally—when I need to focus on God. I love to feel God's voice flow through me.

In 2015, when I retired from my *Living Room* group due to ill health, I was able to continue supporting people with mental health problems by writing for them. But although I love the work, it will never replace the joy of personally sitting at a table with a group sharing the love of Christ.

PLANTING NEW LIVING ROOMS

I once wrote "I'm committed to seeing more *Living Room* groups spring up. I want to see lots of *Living Room*s to serve people who need faith-based support. I want to see this movement securely in place to continue long after I'm gone. Because it's a valuable ministry, a ministry that all Christians with mental illness should have access to. A place where they can talk about both, their faith and mental health issues— probably the only place where they can feel comfortable doing so. I could never give up planting new *Living Rooms*."

This was what I had always believed and worked for. Through my many writings and events like the 100 Huntley Street appearance, the news about *Living Room* spread widely. There was interest, even from a couple as far as South Africa and New Zealand. Quite a few groups were formed in Canada and a couple in the US.

But it was hard to keep it going on my own. Although God had made his presence known and I trusted him, I struggled constantly with bipolar symptoms. Eventually, in July 2014 I was grateful to be able to relinquish care of the *Living Room* ministry and the work of forming new groups to Sanctuary Mental Health Ministries. All I could manage was to continue as facilitator of my own group. For a year I managed to do that until poor mental health made me decide to retire in March of 2015.

CHAPTER FOUR
The Living Room Experience

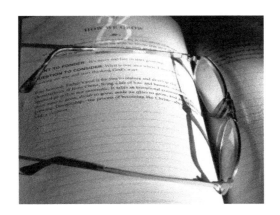

MENTAL HEALTH CHURCH SERVICE

On May 6th, 2007 our church held a mental health service. The event surpassed my expectations.

Speakers from the *Living Room* group spoke openly and from the heart. The congregation was warm and welcoming. They received a hearty applause. The pastor spoke casually and in a compassionate way. He spoke of how we need to look at Jesus in how we live and how we treat others.

It wasn't a sad service at all. All that was discussed was honest and natural. Every now and then there was a wonderful touch of humour. I felt uplifted by it all and I know others did too.

The icing on the cake was the performance of Chalexa's song, *Redeemed*. Chalexa played the piano and Shebee sang.

One neat thing: The pastor mentioned how *Living Room* isn't complete without chocolates. And it's true. Without fail, we have dishes of chocolate on the table at the meetings. We consider it good "medicine." So as people left the sanctuary the pastors' wives served chocolates to them.

As a result of yesterday, a couple of people in the church have indicated they would like to come to the next *Living Room* meeting. This is the great thing about talking so openly about mental health problems: By making it an ok thing to talk about, those who are suffering will feel freer to come into the open and share with others what they are going through. There is no longer a need to keep their pain to themselves. They no longer need to be alone in their struggles, but can find support from people who care.

This is what reducing stigma can do for people. And reducing stigma is possible. Little by little we can do it.

AN AMAZING MEETING

On Friday, May 11, 2007 I wrote:

This afternoon, after the Mental Health Service the *Living Room* meeting had a party atmosphere. So many of us were there. We set up four tables joined to each other to make one huge table that would seat 18 people. My co-facilitator thought I was perhaps overdoing it—and I kind of wondered that as well. Usually we put up three tables which will seat 16. But we ended up with 20 in attendance, an all-time record for us. We had to squeeze a couple of people in on the corners, uncomfortable for them and not something I like to do.

The two ladies who spoke at the service last Sunday told us how they had felt when they shared their story with the congregation. One told us that she had found the experience freeing. Both speakers had received a lot of affirmation after. I know that they were popular after the service ended, with many wanting to speak with them. We celebrated by bringing out a cake with sparklers on it.

Although I'm happy about the success of our support group, I also feel overwhelmed. How long can we continue doing this before it becomes unwieldy? We usually like to have some discussion based on the devotional, but had to forego that today because of lack of time. With ten people in each sharing group, there isn't a lot of time to spare.

I very much want to encourage the formation of more faith-based groups like this and will now have to do some serious work on this. The need is greater than my church and I can adequately respond to. I've decided to write a manual/guide as a tool for churches who wish to do what we have done. But to do a proper job of this I will have to try and get some funding from an organization that shares my vision. I'm working on that.

Please help me pray that I will find a way to spread the *Living Room* concept to other areas. People who suffer from mood disorders need to have a place where they can get support from others who share their faith in God. It is important to have a place where they discuss both: their mental health issues as well as how God works in their life.

THE LIVING ROOM EXPERIENCE

In September 2007 I wrote:

I always came away from *Living Room* meetings with glorious feelings of rejuvenation. When I started facilitating *Living Room* I had never expected that these deep feelings of peace, this holy joy, would be my reward. It's magical. And I have never been more stable or felt as complete as I do after meetings. I know it's because God is truly present at *Living Room*. I'm not leading on my own.

Other members of the group had similar reports. Those two session of *Living Room* each month help them stay well. They learn to cope. They learn to trust God. They learn not to be ashamed of their disorder. And we have a great time together, having lunch, studying scripture, and sharing from our hearts.

I'm encouraged when I hear the stories from members of the group. At one meeting a man and his wife, strong members of their church, had never felt free to talk about his bipolar disorder there. They kept his disorder secret, a burden for which they received no spiritual support. Being able to talk about his problems in the Christian setting we provided gave him tremendous relief. People like this need to have the freedom to share their mental health problems with their church family.

Another *Living Room* member sent the following email. A portion of it read:

"When I told my friend about my support group for mood disorders and what a blessing it was, she asked "isn't it depressing to be around a bunch of crazy people?" I said, "No way, it's a safe place to support each other in our common brokenness and to realize you're not the only one to feel this way. In that setting I've learned that it's an invisible disease in the way some other diseases are. I've learned to dispel the stigma and shame associated with mental illness. My condition is not a curse but could be a blessing. In my lows I get a sense of the emotional pain people can go through."

A STEADY FLAME

To my bloggers on December 29, 2007: I've become lazier than I should be about blogging. There's something about sitting at the computer that doesn't appeal to me these days. Yet there's much I want to share too, and these things keep rolling around in my head.

One thing I've thought a lot of in the last few days is how *Living Room* has become like a steady flame for me, never wavering, never going out. No matter how my mood is, it gives me light. No matter how down I feel, I want to go to the meetings and lead. And no matter how down I feel, I'm *able* to lead. I want to give hope to the people I speak to there, and I always find a source for that hope. What a blessing that is!

In the spring, while I was going through a more severe depression, I thought I'd like to do a favour for a friend. I noticed how that thought was like a spark within me, providing some light, making me feel better. And it felt like that spark lit a candle, one that kept burning for a while. And I thought of how I'd like to share that image with my *Living Room* members. I wanted to tell them how lighting a candle in the dark can help us feel better. Just thinking of sharing this as a devotional kept my candle burning for the rest of the week. I was able to keep my candle lit. I was able to lead a good session.

There were 15 present at yesterday's meeting - not bad for this time of year when most activities are put on hold. We had a wonderful time. I quoted from Philippians 4:6-8 which I've had my Bible lying open to a lot lately:

Do not be anxious about anything, but in everything, by prayer and petition, with thanksgiving, present your requests to God. And the peace of God, which transcends all understanding, will guard your hearts and your minds in Christ Jesus.

After a bit of discussion, we all took turns giving thanks to God. There is truly a peace that comes from thinking of the good things in our lives and being thankful for them. Not only does it help remove anxiety, but it also helps with depression.

At *Living Room* we all support each other. Though I'm the facilitator, I receive support myself as well. I always come away feeling better and—most of the time—feel a wonderful, peaceful kind of joy after. I can be myself there, not having to pretend I'm well when I'm not. Though I'm the leader, I don't have to come across like I've got it all together. In fact, it's better that the members realize that I struggle like they do. When I'm real, everyone is encouraged to be real. There's great beauty in that.

That steady flame that is *Living Room* is an amazing, mysterious thing. It's God at the center. It's made of love. It heals.

EVEN IN A SNOWSTORM

In March 2008 a big snowstorm surprised us on a *Living Room* day. And it was almost April! Snowflakes fell, huge and thick and fast. It was sticking to the grass and to the trees. With all that snow we expected to have a smaller turnout than usual.

We made only thirty cups of coffee instead of the usual thirty-six. Not a good decision, because we ended up with a record turnout of twenty-two. One after another, they kept coming in the door. We pushed five long tables together to make one huge one. Even then, we were packed pretty tight. But we formed a cozy gathering.

We ran out of coffee, we ran out of hot water, we ran out of cold water, and we ran out of meat and veggies. Yet there was plenty other food to eat. Wonderful Cob's buns and Cob's apricot bread. Tillamook cheese, fudge brownies, and much more. No one went hungry.

After introducing the day's topic, "Waiting," and after everyone had thought about it for a while, making notes on their paper, we opened it up for discussion. One member eagerly shared what she was waiting for and amazed us with her story.

Her family had been renting the same house for fourteen years, their kind landlord never raising the rent during that time. Now he was selling the house and they may have to move to more expensive accommodation, something they couldn't afford. They might have to move to a much smaller place that could be cramped for them.

This person's take on it was this, and I'll try to remember what she said:
"I'm excited, looking forward to see what God has in store for us. We may have to move to a two-bedroom apartment, but if we do we'll get triple high bunkbeds. I know everything will work out. I trust what God will do for us, he's always come through in the past. God is good. It will all work out."

This person's faith and trust in God was something to behold. I felt as though we didn't need to go any further with the discussion. But we did, and many people joined in. We all managed to encourage each other.

What we realized was that the important thing when we wait is to keep praying and to partner with God in bringing about a good ending. By praying we are encouraged to have the right attitudes and to live our lives in such a way that we can wait with patience and trust.

AGAPE LOVE AT LIVING ROOM

On February 7, 2009 I was celebrating. Joyous! I'd had a call from a lady in Victoria telling me that her church had its first *Living Room* meeting. Another group was born—the tenth. Praise God!

This particular group will be serving people with all kinds of mental illness, not only mood disorders. It is also not quite ready to do outreach work. Members so far are only from the host church.

I was delighted to hear that the facilitator was genuinely happy about it. And the participants are grateful for the group. They will now have a place where they can be open about both—their faith in God and their mental health issues.

That same day, I wrote this: "Agape love," says theologian Anders Nygren, "Is unmotivated in the sense that it is not contingent on any value or worth in the object of love. It is spontaneous and heedless, for it does not determine beforehand whether love will be effective or appropriate in any particular case."

How I love my *Living Room* group! Even those who seem the most unlovable become very lovable. And in a strange way I come to love the seemingly unlovable even more than those who might seem easier to love. Does that make sense? I thank God for giving me that love for others. Such joy it brings! Yes!

CHAPTER FIVE
Discussion Topics

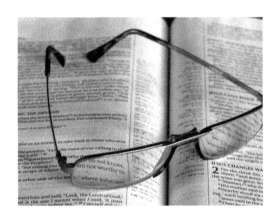

STIGMA, OUR GREATEST ENEMY

From my blog, August 28, 2006:

I want to talk about the topic I'm probably most passionate about/angry about/disgusted with. Although I can speak quite rationally about this, it makes me "mad."

The greatest culprit that stands in the way of the welfare of people living with mental disorders is stigma. Think of how things would be if there were no stigma attached to our disorders:

- we would not have to feel shame
- we would be more willing to accept our illness
- people would be less afraid of giving us support
- we would have higher self-esteem
- we'd be more confident
- we'd be more able to take a significant role in our community
- if our disorders were better accepted, there would be more funds allocated for research
- we'd be more likely to accept medical treatment
- people would be more willing to learn about our disorders so they can support us
- we would not have to feel like outcasts
- there would be less homeless people on the streets
- we would feel more loved
- we would not feel as much pain

The world stigmatizes us. But one of the worst things is that we who live with such disorders accept that stigma. We take it on ourselves. We feel the shame when we shouldn't.

If we could only think of our illness as "just another disease," one that happens to affect our brain... It does not mean we're stupid or that we have bad character. In fact, I believe that people with bipolar disorder are some of the most beautifully sensitive people around. Some of the greatest artists, musicians, and writers were bipolar, and look at what they left the world. Hans Christian Andersen, Frederic Chopin, Lord Byron, Tennessee Williams, Mark Twain, are just a handful of great people who are believed to have had some kind of mood disorder. Even the psalmist, David, had strong moods. Some people, me included, believe that he too could have been bipolar.

LIVING WITHOUT SHAME

On September 26, 2006, I wrote the following in my blog, a topic we talked much about at *Living Room* meetings.

It takes great effort trying to live with confidence when the disorder we have is so stigmatized. It's so utterly unfair that we, who through no fault of our own, have a condition that causes us to hide and live in shame. If you've read some of my earlier posts you will know how angry I am about this.

But what if we were not to feel so ashamed about it? What if we were to recognize how wrong society is about us and say to ourselves, "the heck with them." We know we're okay.

When a person feels he needs to keep something like this secret, it breeds a feeling of shame. How can we possibly win?

I pray that there will be a day when society will be better educated and understanding of what mental illnesses truly are —conditions that happen to affect one of the organs of our body. And it just happens that this organ controls thinking and feelings.

I found a quote recently. Don't know who wrote it but thought someone might be inspired by it:

"If anyone speaks badly of you, live so that none will believe it."

In my own life, I began speaking out about my bipolar disorder ten years ago. I think that writing about it and having a book out helped people respect me. If there are any who think I'm strange because of it, I don't notice it. This has put me at an advantage in many ways. I feel no shame. I only talk about my disorder when there's a reason for doing so. But raising awareness has become more and more my life's work. It is my passion.

I don't know and don't care if people speak badly of me. Maybe some do. But I stubbornly live, being the person God made me to be. Myself.

(Author's Note: But today, in 2020, I'm not sure that being open was the right thing to do. Yes, I ended up raising awareness — in quite a big way. But it was costly. The stigma I fought came back to hurt me deeply in the end.)

UNCOVERING THE GOOD IN THE BAD

On Saturday, May 26, 2007 I wrote the following to a blogging pal:

Living Room was good and left me feeling happy, as all those meetings do. I spent the rest of the day savouring it. After having twenty out to our previous meeting, I decided to make a huge table, pushing five long tables together. That made room for twenty-two chairs to fit around. But only thirteen showed up. Still a good turn-out though.

You won't believe this, Susan, but our topic, "Uncovering the Good in the Bad", was very much like your post about being grateful. We discussed how gratitude can affect how we feel about life and God, and how it affects our mood. Even situations that seem bad at first can eventually give us something to be thankful for if we're in the thanking habit.

In Romans 8:28 Paul said, "*...we know that to those who love God, who are called according to his plan, everything that happens fits into a pattern for good.*"

I told the story about how I'd recently accessed my medical

records from when I was in a mental hospital forty years ago. I'd suspected I had been over-medicated but wanted to be assured of all the facts, since I was writing about it in my latest book. And sure enough, the records show that I had been given excessive amounts of chlorpromazine. My mouth hung open much of the time and I could not communicate with others. There was nothing happening in my brain. It was as though it had stalled.

The part that truly made me bitter was uncovering a letter written by my private psychiatrist's partner, a person who had interviewed me shortly after I was admitted. He had recommended that I be discharged. My previous employer had offered to let me to try and work, despite my psychotic condition. This doctor suggested that I would do better in such a normal environment, rather than a mental institution.

But apparently, this letter was either ignored or not agreed with. I stayed in the hospital for another six interminable months. Miserable months. I was only nineteen years old, the youngest on my ward. It was only when I read these records that I realized this letter existed and that an opportunity had been lost.

I felt stunned and bitter.

But, after a few days, my thinking changed. More than ever before, I began to appreciate how far I had come. I had even more to be thankful for than I realized. God has truly done a lot for me. My records showed that the staff did not hold out much hope for me. My (incorrect) diagnosis was schizophrenia and, in those days, medications were not as effective as they are today. But did I ever show them!!

I'm a fortunate person. And I'm sure that living in the institution in the way I did has benefited me by helping me have compassion and respect for others. I believe what Paul said. If we're in line with God's plan, "...*everything that happens fits into a pattern for good.*" I believe my hospital experiences help me find joy in the work I do with *Living Room*. I'm glad to be a supporter, no longer a victim.

COMPENSATION FOR DEPRESSION

On August 29th, 2007 I wrote the following:

One of my favorite books on depression is *New Light on Depression* by Harold G. Koenig, M.D. and David B. Biebel, D. Min. Much of the book deals with depression from a Christian perspective. I think it's Biebel who said, "...depression's saving grace is not that it can be conquered but that it puts depressed persons of faith in touch with deeper truths about reality, spirituality, and themselves than might otherwise be known." (Yes, I think I understand more about life than those for whom life has been easier.)

He goes on to say—and this is a little bit of a different positive angle I can really relate to:

"Having one's capacity for serenity and joy restored is little compensation for the agony of despair, much less the 'despair beyond despair.' The only true compensation for depression has to do with the sense of purpose and fulfillment that comes from redemptive involvement with others in distress, sharing the comfort we've experienced. This is the true route to joy."

In my own life, I've found a purpose that I probably would not have had, were it not for my bouts with the effects of bipolar disorder, especially the depression. I've come to think of depression as fodder, something bad out of which good can come. Though I suffer as much as anyone while I'm going through it, I know it will help me help others. And helping others *is* "the true route to joy." It truly is.

BATTLE AGAINST SELF-CENTEREDNESS

In February 2007 we had some interesting discussion at *Living Room*.

One thing that had the most impact on me was when someone said how she feels best during depression when she can stop thinking about herself. When she tries to reach out and show an interest in other people's lives, it's easier to forget her own misery. There's something powerful in the act of giving—and that does not only mean giving things, but giving our attention to other people and their stories.

When we're depressed, it's natural to be self-consumed with

misery. In fact, people who suffer from almost any illness are in danger of becoming self-absorbed. It's natural for that to happen.

Interestingly, it's not only a depressed mood that will make us self-absorbed. The same holds true for high moods. When I'm high and I'm with friends, I'll talk their heads off about all the "wonderful" projects I'm engaged in. I totally forget that they have lives too. I forget to ask how they are doing. I'm so full of myself.

But, when I consciously try, and succeed, in asking my friends about themselves: how they're feeling and what they're doing, something happens that makes me feel better about myself. I've come to appreciate having people trust me enough to tell me their troubles. I like the sense of connection it gives us. It feels good to forget about myself.

It's hard, but I must try constantly, to be more other-centered. The payoff is huge. I feel stronger when I reach out. I feel better. I don't feel so much a consumer or victim. I become a contributor and supporter.

Facilitating my *Living Room* support group has helped my emotional well-being in a big way. I feel stronger, more together. Today there are 37 members in the group. Of course, not everyone shows up at the same time. I receive frequent phone calls from people who want to start coming and phone calls from people who want to talk. There are always two or three that need special attention. Serving the needs of these people has given me great joy. I feel I'm doing what God designed me for. *Living Room* has helped me stop thinking of myself overly much. I've prayed for a long time to be more other-centered and *Living Room* has been one of the answers to this prayer.

A blogger made this comment:

> I agree with you 100%. However, I don't agree that we become "Self-Centered." I am so sick and tired of people thinking that those who are depressed or bipolar or who commit suicide are "Selfish" and Self-Centered."
>
> The funny thing is that most people who are depressed or commit suicide tend to keep these things to themselves. They alienate themselves to some degree from life and people. How on earth is that self-centered?
>
> To me, self-centered is similar to Narcissism. They *want* to be centered—they *want* the attention. They *want* everything in life and the world to revolve around them. This is not a description of depression.

DEPRESSION FOR CHRISTIANS

On January 15, 2008, a blogger wrote:

> What are some of your hints to "keep going" when you really feel depressed and just want to stay in bed all day but know that you can't because of family

responsibilities? I take Prozac daily, but because I'm 47 and perimenopausal, I don't think it is working too well at certain times of the month. My kids are 21 (in college), 17 (a senior) and 15...and I can't just lie down and say "out of order today." But that's the way I feel.

By the way, I appreciate your faith-filled posts very much. I sometimes feel guilty that being a Christian I don't always feel or show "the joy of the Lord" because of depressive feelings. And I'm not always that good at hiding them. – Sandy

Dear Sandy,

I think the most important thing you need to remember is that you have an illness and, though it's the nature of depression to make you feel guilty, this is not a justifiable feeling. Christians are not beyond getting depressed, just like they're not beyond having other illnesses. It has nothing to do with your relationship with God and you're not any less of a Christian. Remember that God loves you, no matter what. And there will be times that you will have to allow him to carry you—without feelings of shame or guilt. Just let him take care of you.

Nevertheless, you will feel better if you can manage to do some of the things you would normally do. Even if you do spend a good part of the day in bed, it would be therapeutic to move around and be active off and on through the day.

Why not ask your children or husband to help you with some of the chores? When I've been severely depressed I've found that having my husband help me make dinner or wash the dishes, helped energize me. There's something about working alongside someone that makes the job a lot easier. The social interaction that then happened often boosted my spirit.

In any case, for most people there will be times of brightening—windows of opportunity when you feel like doing more. Take advantage of those windows, but without overdoing it. Eventually you'll have more windows and gradually you will find yourself in a brighter place.

A blogger's comment:

I am a Christian also, and for years I kept feeling like if I just "believed" more or tried harder, the depressive episodes would not exist. Marja's point about how Christians are not exempt from illness (including depression) is so true and FREE-ING!

I found that learning to let go of guilt and remember the message of Christ re: taking his yoke for it is easy and his burden is light. That is such a peaceful verse to me and it reminds me that He knew that there would be a gazillion times in my life where things were just too much.
Also, during depressions, I have found that breaking up large tasks, such as looking at the entire day, became

helpful to me. That is, make a few small goals for the day even if all they are is brushing your teeth and your hair, and then taking a nap.

and treat yourself GENTLY

WHAT WE NEED FOR A LONELY PLACE

On March 2, 2008 I sent out this blog:

Depression is a lonely place to be. The loneliness and disconnectedness we feel must be the worst part of it. We long for someone to reach us through that wall we have around us. We long for love to touch us and bring us out. We long to sense God's presence. We know God loves us, but we can't feel it. We are cold and alone. In limbo.

What can we do to re-connect? How can we find help?

At times like this I long for a call from a friend. I long to hear that someone is thinking of me and praying for me. I long to know that someone cares. That would, I think, in a small way break through the isolation I feel. That would, in a small way, cut through the wall and help me feel some warmth.

I need a friend who will listen to me and just be with me for a while, without making me feel bad about being the way I am. I need a friend who will not tire of sticking with me as I work my way out of the hole I'm in. I need a friend who will love me, no matter how ugly I feel. I need someone I can count on. I need someone who will remind me that God is there.

Comment 1:

Depression is a lonely place, and that is so unfortunate, huh? I mean, there should be more support and to me, there isn't.

I was talking to my mom today and we were talking about some things and her knowing that I am bipolar, she will say how those who are depressed are selfish! I just don't get it.

I know that we've discussed this before within our blogs, but to me, if anything, we are not selfish. How can isolation be selfish? How can feeling so dark and down be selfish?

Comment 2:

Your post has reminded me of my last bad bout with depression which lasted more than a month (a long time for me!).

My husband of 32 years knows just by looking at my face that the darkness is approaching. He is my best friend and at times like that—usually my only friend. My children perceive my depression as "a bad mood" but know it can go on indefinitely.

It is my hope that your husband is a part of your support system at this time.

It is true that I love my Prozac and at those times my dosage is upped in an effort to combat the depression, then tapered back to regular dosage.

My relationship with God becomes all the more closer because I think that only *he* truly understands. He speaks to me all the time—in my mind, in my quiet times, even in my dreams. My husband speaks to me only verbally; he is not inside my head.

I come from a long line of family members who suffered depression and most have attempted and some achieved suicide. For me, suicide is not an option. It is the ultimate separation from God and I never want that.

Growing up with a suicidal parent who didn't think anything of taking his 3 children with him in his attempts using house gas, pills, purposeful car accidents, and fire, the very act of suicide has a different meaning for me personally.

Most people contemplating suicide are surrounded by something they feel is larger than themselves, a situation that cannot be remedied, an abusive person/situation where they see no other way out. Often they feel suicide is the ultimate solution, removing themselves permanently from the problem.

For me, suicide would be taking me away from a place I do not want to be. Instead, because of my life experiences, I choose to turn it around and be more constructive.

I choose to find a way to remove the problem from me, not me from the problem. That may be to cut off a relationship w/person who *is* the problem (temporarily or permanently), to refuse to discuss or to feed into whatever is the root of the problem).

I have even gone so far as to cut ties with family members and friends after repetitive bouts of depression occurred because of them.

MEANING IN THE MIDST OF SUFFERING

March 5, 2008: I have been thinking of why some people who have depression decide they want to die and then take the drastic action to commit suicide. Others with depression— though suffering—choose to live, no matter how dark their life has become. What's the difference? How can we persuade those who want to die that life is worth living? How can we persuade them to choose life, not death? How can we help them find meaning in life?

In 1946, as a result of his experiences as an inmate in a concentration camp, Viktor Frankl wrote a book called *Man's Search for Meaning*. Frankl concludes from his experience that a prisoner's psychological reactions are not solely the result of the conditions of his life, but also from the freedom of choice he always has even in severe suffering. The inner hold a prisoner has on his spiritual self relies on having a faith in the future. Once a prisoner loses that faith, he is doomed.

Frankl quotes Nietzsche: "He who has a *why* to live for can bear with almost any *how*."

We who live with the highs and lows of bipolar disorder can learn from this. We know that we're going to hit depressions. Depression for us is unavoidable. What we need to do is to create a life for ourselves that is meaningful. During the times we're well we can build purpose into our lives, purpose that will be so important to us that we will hang on to the hope it gives, even during times of depression. We can choose to create a life for ourselves that will be so rewarding that we would not want to lose it, no matter how difficult the struggle becomes.

Personally, I have found meaning in facilitating *Living Room*. Now when I get depressed, I try to learn from what I'm going through so that I can share insights with members of the group. Even the bad stuff has value in it, though it may at the time be difficult to see. I know that this is God's work I'm doing and I have faith that he will help me do it, even when things get tough.

Everyone has gifts they can use to create a rich life for themselves, one they would never want to give up. But we have to work on building that kind of life while we are well.

GIVING SUPPORT

July 3, 2008: Earlier this week a blogger wrote about the importance of wanting wellness if we want to be well. "As far as I am concerned, the most critical component of achieving wellness is wanting it....Wellness doesn't occur in a vacuum. Whether or not you believe that bipolarity and/or clinical depression is a biochemical condition, the only way to achieve wellness is to be willing to ask the difficult questions, and live a life that matters."

I wrote a comment expressing my frustrations with someone I'm giving support to who doesn't seem to want that wellness. At least she doesn't pursue it as I wish she would. I wondered at what point I should back off. My blogging pal followed her initial post with one she titles *When to Let Go*. She talks about her feelings on the issue: "So, I guess my answer is that I believe the woman you're talking about needs to find professional help. And she needs to 'step up to the plate' so to speak. If you continue to allow her to take from you, you'll have nothing left. And if she decides that life isn't worth living, ultimately that's her decision."

But, when I think back to what I felt like when I was depressed, and how difficult it was to be well, and how important it was for me to have the people I loved not give up on me, I can't see myself giving up on others. Perhaps backing off a bit and not staying too close is good for my own health, but I feel I need to stay available.

In his book, *New Light on Depression*, Harold Koenig wrote some things that I have taken to heart. He wrote: "Love—unconditional love—is the ultimate long-term antidote for depression, for at its core love is connected with faith and hope."

I feel that we need to always remind people they are loved and not withdraw that love from people when they're going through hard times. One of the most important things a person with depression needs is to know that there's someone always available. Knowing that someone is available who understands—because she's been there herself—is invaluable.

Since starting *Living Room*, I've given support to quite a few people. While it isn't easy, it can be rewarding too. Though I walk with them through their valleys, I also experience with them the relief when they climb out again. When they call me and spend some time expressing their feelings to me and I have no answers, we can always turn to God at the end of the call. When I feel helpless and don't know what to say, we pray together. And those prayers are powerful. I feel the presence of God's Spirit.

We call on God to give the person strength and patience. We ask him to embrace her and to help her feel his love. We turn everything over to God. When we hang up I feel I can leave it all behind because it's in God's hands, not mine. This is how I can usually manage to support people without it getting myself down.

As a Christian I need to be a conduit of Christ's love. And I've found that it's a joy to be that. It's rewarding to be that. And to walk with someone through their depression—to talk with them and to help them go to God with it—is a privilege.

I don't expect that everyone should be able to do this. I don't judge people who are not able to do this. We all have gifts that make us unique. This just happens to be mine.

TRUST

In my blog on September 10, 2008 I wrote the following. At *Living Room* we will be talking about trust. Being able to trust in God, to trust our ability to be well, to trust our doctor, and so on. It's important to a life of peace. It's important to our health.

When I start getting symptoms that indicate a depression might be coming on, I need to trust that it won't happen. When I trust and rely on God to help me avert it, I have a much greater chance of staying well. Someone—and I'm too lazy right now to check the source—once said that when we fear God we need fear nothing else. "Fearing God" meaning to believe in God and his power—to be in awe of God.

To have bipolar disorder can bring on a lot of fears because we have had so many bad experiences with depression, mania and psychosis. The slightest indication that something is going wrong can bring on anxiety, making it even more likely that it will.

In Matthew 6:25-34, Jesus speaks poetically: "*Therefore I tell you, do not worry about your life, what you will eat or drink; or about your body, what you will wear....Who of you by worrying can add a single hour to his life?*"...(I won't type out the entire piece.) But then Jesus says, "*But seek first his kingdom and his righteousness, and all these things will be given to you as well.*"

Jesus is not saying that we will have immunity to the problems of life, but by trusting God instead of ourselves, we will have confidence in spite of them. When we seek the kingdom of God we will find purpose, power and direction. We forget about being anxious. We trust where God is taking us. It's through faith, hope and extending God's love to others - as God loves us - that we will experience this kingdom of God - this kingdom where God's rule prevails.

LOVE AND THE PAIN OF SUICIDE

In September 2009 I gave a talk to a suicide loss group. It was an emotionally charged time with twenty-one of us sitting in a circle for three hours. They shared with me their stories of pain at losing someone to suicide. There were many tears. I deeply felt their grief. The emotions stayed with me for a long time.

I told them what it's like to live with bipolar disorder and what it's like to be so depressed that you want to die. I shared honestly, totally myself, transparent.

Although this was a secular group I did tell them a bit about my faith and how it helps me survive. About how I need God. How could I not? But I did not dwell on it too much. We needed to address their feelings more than anything.

They were grateful to me for sharing and I was just as grateful to them for their sharing. I needed to hear and see the kind of pain they were suffering because there have been times when I have considered suicide. I needed to hear how their lives were forever changed by their losses. I don't want to do that to the people I love.

God, when I'm depressed, please help me remember the pain I could cause to those who love me. Though it may be hard, help me know that people love me, though my depression might tell me otherwise.

I prayed for God's presence before I went to the meeting last night and he *was* there. His love was there in that circle. He was amongst us.

HOW MUCH WE'RE LOVED!

I learned something from the suicide loss group that I wish I could broadcast everywhere.

I don't think any of us realize how much we're loved. Especially not when we're depressed and our perspective is off. Even when we're told we are loved, we tend not to believe it.

Yet the love those twenty-one people expressed for the children, spouses and parents they lost showed me how deeply those who died were loved. And those who died may not have been aware. What a tragedy! The survivors in the circle probably didn't even realize how deeply they could love and how much pain they could suffer.

I believe we love our family and friends far more deeply than we know. The busyness of our lives tends to distract us from what's important. We get so busy focusing on activities and "stuff" that we forget to consider our appreciation for each other. We might be forgetting to tell our loved ones how much they mean to us. And we so need to do that.

My husband and I came face to face with what this might mean for him, were I to take my life, as I had wanted to in the past. I came to see the incredible pain it would cause him. And he recognized how he can't take me for granted. He saw how real such a loss could be. And me? I would never want to inflict such pain.

I pray to God that I will never be so self-centered that I will forget what I learned....And yet, the reality of it is that when such emotional pain comes it's pretty hard to think beyond it.

AND YET...

On April 20, 2010, we studied Psalms 42 and 43 at our *Living Room* Bible study. It sure hit home for those of us there. We could relate to the psalmists' laments. We could relate for the thirsting after God expressed in the opening verses:

"As the deer pants for streams of water,
so my soul pants for you, O God.
My soul thirsts for God, for the living God.
When can I go and meet with God?"

You'll remember the wonderful hymn based on this Psalm. How well that song ministered to me a few weeks ago when a friend shared it with me!

As we studied these Psalms we saw how the writers expressed their depression, but clung to the hope they had in God. Despite everything, they're able to say,

"Put your hope in God,
for I will yet praise him,
my Savior and my God."

Oh to be able to cling to God in that way! Despite everything, to be able to say *"...I will yet praise him."*

These same words are repeated three times within Psalm 42 and 43.

How can we who suffer from mood disorders hang onto such faith? How can we get ourselves to the place where we can say, "…and yet I will praise him. In spite of everything, I will praise him."

I think we need to keep wanting God, to keep hungering for him. We need to talk to him. And that can start by simply saying "hello" to him. I believe God is pleased when we yearn for him and he will be there for us. He will show Himself. The Bible says that he who seeks will find. So true!!

God is always there. He doesn't leave; it's we who leave him.

CHAPTER SIX
The Importance of Faith

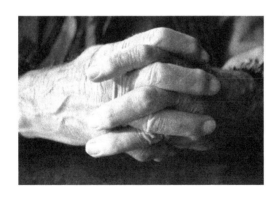

LIVING ROOM'S FOCUS ON FAITH

The *Living Room* ministry I founded in 2006 pioneered the combination of faith with mental health as a form of helping people deal with their mental health challenges. It introduced the church to the important role it could play in the well-being of those who struggle with mental health issues.

From the beginning, *Living Room* groups were faith-based. That meant that the biggest part of our focus was faith—faith in how God can help us cope and manage our difficult lives. A good portion of our meetings—at least 30 minutes—was dedicated to reflecting on Scripture and what it could teach us about our mental health difficulties. The Bible is rich. The Psalms alone can encourage and comfort us in the many ups and downs we experience.

I myself had learned years earlier how important it was to be able to trust God and to be assured of his never-ending love. Although I didn't find complete healing of my disorder, I learned that I could count on a *measure* of healing.

When I led *Living Room* I learned to understand the kinds of messages people with depression and anxieties should be hearing. I saw how learning about Jesus, the friend of outcasts, helped them realize they were like today's outcasts. Jesus spent time with these people, not unlike themselves, showing his acceptance and love. This knowledge comforted them. They realized that with God, they are as worthy anyone else.

Individuals living with mental health challenges hunger for God. They need to be spiritually fed by those who themselves have such challenges—people who understand them, people who know Jesus Christ.

In 2013 I started writing devotionals specifically for individuals with mental health challenges. When I could no longer lead a group, I was able to send them out via email and blog. This is how I continued my ministry.

SPIRITUAL INFLUENCE ON MENTAL HEALTH

In September 2007, I wrote the following to my blogging pals:

I've been meaning for a while to draw from Harold Koenig's book, *Faith & Mental Health*, and share with you some of the treasures of thinking and understanding I have found there.

Koenig tells of nearly 500 studies during the twentieth century that reported statistically significant associations between religion and mental health. (478 out of 724 studies) (page 133)

He lists and explains ten ways in which religion could improve mental health. Religion:

1. Promotes a positive worldview
2. Helps to make sense of difficult situations
3. Gives purpose and meaning
4. Discourages maladaptive coping
5. Enhances social support
6. Promotes other-directedness
7. Helps to release the need for control
8. Provides and encourages forgiveness
9. Encourages thankfulness
10. Provides hope.

I wish I had the room here and the time to go into each of these points in detail. What will have to suffice is my testimony that I have found all these important in my Christian walk and important in my ability to be well. Not that I'm always perfectly well. Those who have come to know me will remember many times I have struggled. Yet my faith has grown and my mental health has improved since I began following Christ. I love my life. God has given me much to be grateful for.

Good, non-judgmental Christian support is important for those who suffer from mental illness. People with such illnesses need Christ-like love, so they will be encouraged in their faith—so they will benefit from their faith.

STIGMA IN THE CHURCH

Written in October 2007:

Why don't people within the church feel comfortable discussing mental health issues?

I think a major reason is that people don't understand mental illness enough to be able to talk about it. They need education. The problem is, sometimes they don't want to be educated. Often it is fear. People fear what they don't understand and they can't get beyond the block that creates.

In churches and in Christian writings the reason for emotional problems has frequently been attributed to spiritual problems. A person attending a *Living Room* group recently told us of how—when she told her pastor that she was being treated for depression—he told her to "praise the Lord and you will feel better." Instead of receiving compassion, he gave her the message that all she needed to do was to turn to God. In other words, if her relationship with God was better, she would not be depressed. It was as though he was blaming her for the depression.

Illnesses like depression are too often not recognized as the diseases they are. If the problem is emotional it is believed that it is within your own power to change. If the problem is within our mind, it is believed to be our own fault. People have trouble understanding that the brain is an organ and, like any other organ of our body, something can go wrong with it. This affects our feelings, our thinking, and our behavior. This is what people—especially Christians—need to understand.

How are we going to change this faulty thinking?

I think it would help for church congregations to hear testimonies from people with mental illness. They need to hear illustrations of the medical nature of their disease. They need to hear that people can be good Christians while, at the same time, dealing with mental health issues.

Stigma within the church is the most damaging, more so than stigma within secular society. This is because a person's faith in God comes into question. When a person is struggling with mental illness, the worst thing for him to hear is that his relationship with God is at fault or that it's the devil causing his emotional turmoil.

The church, as the body of Christ with its message of his unconditional love, is in the best position to help people with mental illness. Christians are in the best position to give Christ-like support. This is the kind of support we who suffer expect from the church. This kind of support will help us keep the faith we so badly need. But Christians need to educate themselves; they need to learn to understand; they need to be compassionate and not judge.

A blogger responding to this said:

> I can tell you that it isn't much better in the Jewish faith. I
> have bipolar disorder, mild schizophrenia, and epilepsy.
> None of these are ever to be discussed within my
> household. They are all stigmas that get swept under the
> carpet, hushed up and never spoken about. Even my
> epilepsy, a true medical malady (if you don't buy the fact
> that bipolar disorder is a disease) is not spoken about.
> There is something wrong with a person who has seizures
> that is taboo. The women in my family, the Jewish
> gossipers, they love to whisper about it, but it is not
> something that is learned or discussed by members of the
> family...setting my life back about 200 years.

MENTAL ILLNESS: HOW CAN CONGREGATIONS RESPOND?

In March 2011, canadianchristianity.com asked me to write
on this topic.

PART 1

A friend emailed me about an acquaintance who had been
newly diagnosed with bipolar illness. Bill had struggled and
suffered a lot in the previous years with undiagnosed severe
depression. Although the bipolar diagnosis was hard to live
with, he realized that he needed to accept it and learn to
manage it. Writes my friend, "He has encountered much
condemnation and misjudgment from his church and

Christian friends." This is very discouraging because he knows how important a supportive church is if he is to walk closely with the Lord. Now he is looking for a church where people will accept him and love him with Christ's unconditional love so he can grow together with them.

This kind of story—and I have heard many of them—disturbs me deeply because I too have bipolar disorder. I can identify with this man and so know the need for understanding and compassion. I too struggle to manage my illness and often falter. In spite of good medications, I still have times when my strong moods break through and I suffer severely.

But I am fortunate. I have a church that is accepting, with good friends and a pastor who has come to understand bipolar disorder. They support me through those many times when I'm up or down. My friends have learned about my disorder through reading and through what I have told them about it. Although they'll never fully understand what I go through, they try. I can talk to them and they encourage me, not trying to fix me, realizing that I'm doing the best I can. Thanks to them I have received the kind of unconditional love that Bill yearns for. They are enabling me to grow with them and, in turn, they grow with me.

How I wish it could be so for everyone who suffers from mental illness! The need for acceptance is great. The need to be encouraged in their faith is great.

People with mental illnesses like bipolar, schizophrenia, anxiety, and depression need a healing of their whole person —their mind, body and spirit. They need care physically (including medical care), psychologically (perhaps including counselling), and spiritually through worship, prayer, and Bible study with others.

The church and educated Christian friends are in the best position to help fellow Christians in their struggles with mental health problems. It's not easy, as any of you who have had to deal with mentally ill people will know. And with one in five people at some time of their life suffering from a mental illness, most of you will have had some experience trying to be supportive in some way. Although I do relatively well with my bipolar disorder, I know it isn't always easy on my husband and friends. The effects of my ups and downs can be hard on them. But I'm hoping they have been rewarded by having seen me blossom into someone who is now able to help others.

With the encouragement of my pastor and friends I was able to start a peer support ministry we call *Living Room*. Through the website and manuals we have helped other people with mood disorders start groups in their own churches. Now there are at least eleven groups helping people with depression, anxiety and bipolar disorders receive Christian support. This is one way churches can help.

Another valuable thing would be to have sermons occasionally referring to mental health issues and the needs of those who are mentally ill. When congregations hear their pastors speak openly about it, they will in turn feel freer to be open about problems they themselves or family members and friends might be having. The important thing is to make mental illness an okay thing to talk about, taking away feelings of shame.

Yes, I'm fortunate. I receive the benefit of loving support from my congregation. But there are many who don't. For them, the stigma is sometimes worse than the disorder itself. Will your church offer people like Bill or me a spiritual home? Will you offer us the Christian support we so desperately need?

In part two, I will show how Christians can give practical help to friends who are suffering from mental health problems.

MENTAL ILLNESS: HOW CAN CONGREGATIONS RESPOND?

PART 2

Christians who try to help a friend with mental illness need to remember how Job's friends treated him and learn from that story. In his introduction to the book of Job in *The Message*, Eugene Peterson wrote, "The moment we find ourselves in trouble of any kind—sick in the hospital, bereaved by a friend's death, dismissed from a job or relationship, depressed or bewildered—people start showing up telling us exactly what is wrong with us and what we must do to get better...More often than not, these people use the Word of God frequently and loosely. They are full of spiritual diagnosis and prescription...But then we begin to wonder, 'Why is it that for all their apparent compassion we feel worse instead of better after they've said their piece?'"

Job's friends were judgmental, trying to find ways of blaming Job for his afflictions. One friend said, "Oh that Job might be tested to the utmost for answering like a wicked man! To his sin he adds rebellion; scornfully he claps his hands among us and multiplies his words against God." (Job 34:36-37) Here is how God responded to this friend: "I am angry with you and your two friends, because you have not spoken of me what is right, as my servant Job has." (Job 42:7) Job had been honest with God. Perhaps his friends would have been more helpful by entering with him in his suffering and helping him look for God.

Can you love a friend with depression or other major mental illness, realizing he has a disorder of the brain that is not his fault? Can you show compassion without suggesting easy answers? Can you encourage without trying to advise or fix? Can you listen without making light of a pain that runs deep? That's the non-judgmental way. That's the caring way. Mostly what we who live with mental illness need is for someone to care enough to listen and have empathy. Isn't that all Job wanted and needed?

What are some practical things you can do to help a friend with depression? There are many. They're similar to what you would do to help physically ill people. You might bring them a casserole. You might give them a call once in a while, telling them you're thinking of them and praying for them. You would ask them how their day is going. We who live with mental illness need the same things. We might need a ride to the doctor or help shopping for groceries. A reminder of scripture that might have helped you yourself during trials could help. Going for a walk with us would be therapeutic. A hug now and then could do wonders.

At times I feel ashamed for things I've done or how I've reacted to situations. Then it's hard to live with myself. Then I need Christ's unconditional love, shown to me through my friends. It's then that I need to be reminded that God forgives. I need to be reminded that everyone is broken in some way, even when they don't have a mental disorder.

This is Christ-like giving at its best. This kind of care gives me comfort. And when—through my friends—I receive God's comfort in this way, I am able to comfort others who suffer as I do. (2 Corinthians 1:3-4)

My prayer is that others who live with mental illnesses will receive the kind of care I've received from my Christian friends. My prayer is that Christians will learn more about mental health issues and how to support those who suffer emotionally. There are many of us and we need you.

APPENDIX ONE
Interactive Devotionals for Meetings

DEVOTIONAL 1. AVOIDING ISOLATION

The solitary confinement that prisoners are sometimes put through as punishment is cruel. Yet the emotional isolation experienced in depression is a similar prison, one not easily escaped.

- How can we avoid the isolation we experience during depression?
- How can we trust and wait patiently for the depression to lift?

Nelson Mandela, in his autobiography, *Die Wit Man*, wrote about his experience with solitary confinement:

"I was locked up for 23 hours a day, with 30 minutes of exercise in the morning and again in the afternoon... There was no natural light in my cell; a single bulb burned overhead 24 hours a day...I had nothing to read, nothing to write on or with, no one to talk to. The mind begins to turn in on itself, and one desperately wants something outside of oneself on which to fix one's attention. I have known men who have taken half-a-dozen lashes in preference to being locked up alone."

Mandela went on to talk about the relief brought about when an insect appeared from the crack in the floor and he had something he could watch – something to keep him company and preoccupy him.

Being deeply depressed could be looked on as emotional solitary confinement.

- How is deep depression like Mandela's experience in solitary confinement?
- How can we find relief, the way Mandela did in watching the insect? What are the simple pleasures that help you with your sense of isolation?
- But when our depression is not deep or when we are only on the verge of a depression, what strategies can we employ to avoid isolation?
- How can we reach beyond ourselves? to others? to God?

The psalmist, David, knew about isolation. The following psalm is something many of us will be able to relate to. David often talks about his fear of going down into the pit, but he always ends by expressing his trust in God's love and protection. We can hang onto God's great love for us, knowing he will always be there for us.

How long, O Lord? Will you forget me forever?
How long will you hide your face from me?
How long must I wrestle with my thoughts
and every day have sorrow in my heart?
How long will my enemy triumph over me?
Look on me and answer, O Lord my God.
Give light to my eyes, or I will sleep in death;

But I trust in your unfailing love;
my heart rejoices in your salvation.
I will sing to the Lord,
for he has been good to me.

Psalm 13:1-3, 5-6

In her book *The Hiding Place*, Corrie ten Boom includes a wonderful line:

"There is no pit so deep that God's love is not deeper still."

DEVOTIONAL 2. CONSIDER IT PURE JOY...

...whenever you face trials

Consider it a sheer gift, friends, when tests and challenges come at you from all sides. You know that under pressure, your faith-life is forced into the open and shows its true colors. So don't try to get out of anything prematurely. Let it do its work so you become mature and well-developed, not deficient in any way. (James 1:2-4 MSG)

• What kinds of hardships have you had to face?
• Did you find them to be a gift—a joy?
• How could a trial be a gift?

Consider it pure joy, my brothers and sisters, whenever you face trials of many kinds, because you know that the testing of your faith produces perseverance. Let perseverance finish its work so that you may be mature and complete, not lacking anything. (James 1:2-4 NIV))

God is constantly trying to teach us how dependent we are on Him, that we are held completely in his hands, reliant on his care alone. We need to show that we won't try to take a step on our own. We must stand on God's strength, not our own.

- How have you learned to rely on God through what you've suffered?
- What makes faith easier to learn through trials than through an easy life?

These trials will show that your faith is genuine. It is being tested as fire tests and purifies gold--though your faith is far more precious than mere gold. So when your faith remains strong through many trials, it will bring you much praise and glory and honor on the day when Jesus Christ is revealed to the whole world. (1 Peter 1:7 NLT)

See, I have refined you, though not as silver;
I have tested you in the furnace of affliction (Isaiah 48:10 NIV)

- In what ways do you feel God has helped you survive your trials?
- How has God refined you through your trials? Do you feel you're a better person for having suffered?

- Would you consider it "pure joy" to suffer trials?

We will close with the way we started:

Consider it a sheer gift, friends, when tests and challenges come at you from all sides. You know that under pressure, your faith-life is forced into the open and shows its true colors. So don't try to get out of anything prematurely. Let it do its work so you become mature and well-developed, not deficient in any way. (James 1:2-4 MSG)

What a Great God we have who will use even our hardships to make us better people.

DEVOTIONAL 3. COPING WITH ANXIETY

When we're anxious we usually take very shallow breaths, cutting down on the oxygen level in our brain. This lack of oxygen will make you feel out of control, not able to solve the problems you might be facing. Breathing deeply will calm your brain and help you feel more relaxed.

When you feel anxiety coming on, change your breathing. Take a deep breath through your nose, hold it, and then let it go out through your mouth.

When you breathe in, you're gathering strength. When you breathe out, you will relax.

In my CBT anxiety class we learned to use coping statements while we do this breathing. We repeat the same statement whenever we need to do our breathing. When we get tired of one statement, we try another one.

The following are some coping statements:

- I can ride this through - I don't need to let this get to me
- I have survived this before and I can survive this time, too.
- I will use my coping skills and allow this to pass.
- Anxiety will not hurt me, even if it does not feel good.

But I've found something that works even better. By making my coping statement a Bible verse or part of a verse, I encourage myself—not only psychologically—but spiritually. I'm turning to God, trusting Him to help me get over my fears. In the process I draw closer to him. Every time I breathe and repeat a coping verse to myself, I'm practising his presence.

BIBLICAL COPING STATEMENTS

You will want to find your own favourite verses to use, but here are a few to get you started:

- *The Lord is my shepherd, I lack nothing.*
  He makes me lie down in green pastures, (Psalm 23:1-2)
- *Cast all your anxiety on him because he cares for you.* (1Peter 5:7)

- *"Be still, and know that I am God;"* (Psalm 46:10)
- *Do not be anxious about anything, but in everything, by prayer and petition, with thanksgiving, present your requests to God.* (Philippians 4:6)
- *I can do everything through him who gives me strength.* (Philippians 4:13)
- *"My grace is sufficient for you, for my power is made perfect in weakness."* (2 Corinthians 12:9)
- *"Never will I leave you; never will I forsake you."* (Hebrews 13:5)
- *With God all things are possible...* (Matthew 19:26)
- *"Come to me, all you who are weary and burdened, and I will give you rest.* (Matthew 11:28)
- *[Nothing] will be able to separate us from the love of God...* (Romans 8:39)

DEVOTIONAL 4. DAVID: A MAN OF COURAGE AND STRENGTH

Courage and strength—and where we get it from—is a huge topic and in preparing this devotional I got quite overwhelmed. Where should I start?

Then I thought of David, one of my favourite characters in the Bible. Maybe if we study him we can get a clue to where we ourselves could get courage and strength from.

- Can you relate to David in any way? How?

David had a huge amount of courage because he trusted that God would be with him and protect him. Look at the courage he had as a youth when he slew Goliath, the Philistine giant. Behold his attitude in 1 Samuel 17:32-36:

David said to Saul: Let no one lose heart on account of this Philistine; your servant will go and fight him."

Saul replied, "You are not able to go out against this Philistine and fight him; you are only a boy, and he has been a fighting man from his youth."

But David said to Saul, "Your servant has been keeping his father's sheep. When a lion or a bear came and carried off a sheep from the flock, I went after it, struck it and rescued the sheep from its mouth. When it turned on me, I seized it by its hair, struck it and killed it. Your servant has killed both the lion and the bear; this uncircumcised Philistine will be like one of them, because he has defied the armies of the living God.

I like where he said "because [the Philistine] has defied the armies of the Living God." That to me shows where his courage came from.

• Do you see it?

David said to the Philistine, "You come against me with sword and spear and javelin, but I come against you in the name of the Lord Almighty, the God of the armies of

Israel, whom you have defied. This day the Lord will hand you over to me, and I'll strike you down and cut off your head. Today I will give the carcasses of the Philistine army to the birds of the air and the beasts of the earth, and the whole world will know that there is a God in Israel. (1 Samuel 17:45-46)

In his mind David thinks, "How dare they defy our God?" He was angry and, with God so much a part of whom he was, the anger gave him courage and strength.

Each of us has a Goliath in our life. Probably several. For those of us here, a mental health problem is one of them. It takes courage and strength to overcome it—to survive and thrive, to live a productive life. When our hearts and minds are set on God—when we trust Him—he will help us.

- Think of situations when God helped you and gave you courage and strength.

If you look up passages in your Bible dealing with strength— and there are many—you will be encouraged to note that it is not *your* strength that is needed but the strength that God supplies.

Trust that God will give you strength and you will receive it.

Philippians 4:13 - *I can do everything through him who gives me strength.*

DEVOTIONAL 5. GIVING THANKS IN ALL CIRCUMSTANCES

1 THESSALONIANS

In this letter Paul was addressing real issues with the Thessalonians—their morality, their love for one another, their fears. But he expresses himself in a spirit of thankfulness.

We give thanks to God always for all of you, constantly mentioning you in our prayers. (1 Thessalonians 1:2)

And we also thank God constantly for this, that when you received the word of God, which you heard from us, you accepted it not as the word of men but as what it really is, the word of God, which is at work in you believers. (1 Thessalonians 2:13)

For what thanksgiving can we return to God for you, for all the joy that we feel for your sake before our God. (1 Thessalonians 3:9)

Be joyful always; pray continually; give thanks in all circumstances, for this is God's will for you in Christ Jesus. (1 Thessalonians 5:16-18)

• Are you able to give thanks in all circumstances?

If you look closely, you'll see that Paul is not telling you to be thankful *for* troubling circumstances. Rather, we are to be thankful *in* our circumstances. There is a major difference between being thankful *for* every situation in life and being thankful *in* those situations.

- Is it possible to be thankful while depressed?
- How can we develop a spirit of thankfulness?

Being thankful in all circumstances requires consistent listening to God's promises and looking for God's goodness toward our lives. Maybe our attention is turned inward on ourselves. We grumble and complain.

Complaining is a symptom of an unthankful heart. It isn't the product of a deprived life. Giving a child everything he wants results in an ungrateful child. He feels he's entitled to everything and wants more. He's never satisfied – never happy.

Thankfulness isn't the result of having a lot. Christians in Uganda are thankful for the smallest kindness, and they sing with a joy that would put our singing to shame. It flows from a heart that sees and hear God's goodness. They are listening to God's promises.

We need to hear promises like:

And we know that for those who love God all things work together for good, for those who are called according to his purpose. (Romans 8:28)

Does this mean we can't be honest about our problems?

- Does than mean we should never tell a friend when something is wrong with us or bothering us?
- Does that mean we can't share our problems here at *Living Room*?

To have close relationships with friends we need to be able to share honestly. If we're not authentic our friendships will be plastic. We shouldn't be afraid to say something about a deep concern or problem. *Living Room* will only be helpful if we can be honest about what we are going through. We trust in God's presence and bring everything to him in prayer.

I have a friend who tells me the problems she's having but invariably will end by saying "But God is good." It's a bit like how David wrote his psalms isn't it? Look at Psalm 13 for example. He's obviously in a desperate state and complaining to God. And yet he ends with:

But I trust in your unfailing love;
my heart rejoices in your salvation.
I will sing to the Lord,
for he has been good to me.

Expect the good, expect blessings. Look for what is good and you will find it. There's a huge benefit to having a grateful spirit. It brings joy and helps keep depression at bay.

APPENDIX TWO
More about Living Room

CHRISTIAN PEER SUPPORT

Peer support groups like Living Room are an important element in the needs of those living with mental health issues. Support by peers has been shown to be more effective than support from healthy individuals.

According to Phyllis Solomon, PhD from the University of Pennsylvania, peer support "is viewed as a more active approach to coping with illness, promoting choice and self-determination that enhance empowerment, as opposed to the passivity engendered by "participation in services with a hierarchical structure."

Christian groups like Living Room are vitally important. There are few other places where a group of individuals with mental illness can gather to talk about both: their emotional struggles and their trust in God. Those who don't have lived experience can't hope to empathize in the way peers can.
Being part of a faith-based group like Living Room helps participants in several ways. They receive social support, support coping with their mental health, and enrichment of their faith life.

Churches and the people with lived experience who attend need to grow in awareness about Christian peer support and its value. Those who might consider leading a group like Living Room will have to be able to count on their church for encouragement and support. Facilitators will need training.

The church has made great strides in the acceptance and support of those living with mental illness. But if faith-based peer support groups are not made available, the very people they're trying to help might be missing out on the best support of all—the support they can give each other.

WHY WE NEED FAITH-BASED PEER SUPPORT

Individuals living with mental health issues need peer support like Living Room where they can support others who know what it is to have such issues. They can give the kind of support healthy individuals can seldom provide. They can encourage each other through Christ to be the best they can be.

What kind of support can a peer support group offer that isn't available elsewhere?

- Those who have suffered with mental illness can best testify to how God helped them.
- They can have more compassion than those who don't know what mental ill health feels like.
- They can encourage each other's faith through sharing experiences.
- Members can encourage each other to see themselves as people like others, not to be looked down on.
- They could learn to be a stronger person: a victor of their disease rather than a victim.
- They can learn how to do more than just receive support; they can give it too.

• Members are reminded that their illness is not who they are. It's what they deal with.
• Members can freely discuss their struggles without feelings of guilt or shame.
• They can help each other overcome the effects of stigma.
• They can pray for each other.
• They will know they're not alone. Others suffer as they do but are able to be contributing members of the community.

HUNGER FOR GOD

Those who have mental health problems are hungry for God. If they're going to find wholeness, this hunger needs to be fed. I know this from my own life experience. And I know it from the times I've spent in psychiatric facilities. Patients were unashamedly open to reveal their need. Eager to embrace the thought of a God who loves them.

THE EFFECTIVENESS OF GROUP PEER SUPPORT

Five theoretical frameworks have been used in attempts to explain the effectiveness of self-help groups.
Solomon, Phyllis (2004). "Peer support/peer provided services underlying processes, benefits, and critical ingredients". Psychiatric Rehabilitation Journal.

1. Social support: Having a community of people to give physical and emotional comfort, people who love and care, is a moderating factor in the development of psychological and physical disease.

2. Experiential knowledge: Members obtain specialized information and perspectives that other members have obtained through living with severe mental illness. Validation of their approaches to problems increase their confidence.

3. Social learning theory: Members with experience become creditable role models.

4. Social comparison theory: Individuals with similar mental illness are attracted to each other in order to establish a sense of normalcy for themselves. Comparing one another to each other is considered to provide other peers with an incentive to change for the better either through upward comparison (looking up to someone as a role model) or downward comparison (seeing an example of how debilitating mental illness can be).

5. Helper theory: Those helping each other feel greater interpersonal competence from changing other's lives for the better. The helpers feel they have gained as much as they have given to others. The helpers receive "personalized learning" from working with "helpees." The helpers' self-esteem improves with the social approval received from those they have helped, putting them in a more advantageous position to help others.

LEADING IN THE NAME OF JESUS

HOW TO BE A HUMBLE LEADER

Have this mind among yourselves, which is yours in Christ Jesus, who, though he was in the form of God, did not count

equality with God a thing to be grasped, but emptied himself, by taking the form of a servant, being born in the likeness of men.
Philippians 2:5-7

Years ago when I was training Living Room facilitators, my favourite resource was Henri Nouwen's book, *In the Name of Jesus: Reflections on Christian Leadership*. Although it was published in 1989, years before Living Room got its start, the book contains wonderful lessons for those leading support groups. It would be good for all Christian leaders to read.

Nouwen was a Catholic priest with an interest in using psychology as a means of exploring the human side of faith – something he felt was being overlooked from a pastoral standpoint. The reason I believe many of us may identify with him is because he suffered from depression as so many of us do. He is an ideal person to teach us about faith-based support leadership for people with mental health issues.

One of the greatest dangers in leadership is pride. The desire to look self-assured can cause us to present ourselves as wiser and closer to God than those we lead. Unintentionally we might set ourselves above others in the group. But this is not the kind of leader a peer support group should have. Every member, even the leader, should be a peer—an equal. Humility is of utmost importance.

According to Nouwen, leaders need to show their own woundedness instead of feigning more wholeness than is theirs to show. Says Nouwen: "We are not the givers of life. We are sinful, broken, vulnerable people who need as much care as anyone we care for." (p. 61-62) This is especially true when leading a peer support group.

"The servant leader is a vulnerable servant who needs the people as much as they need their leader." (p. 63)

Through modelling vulnerability and candidly revealing pain and insecurities, facilitators can encourage the entire group to do the same. Honestly sharing faith and doubt, hope and despair, joy and sadness with others helps bring members of the group in touch with God. They need to get the message that there's no need for shame.

Most members of Living Room groups have suffered or are suffering. It's this commonality that pulls them together as a group, jointly drawing them closer to Jesus. We learn to fellowship with each other and the suffering Christ.

Jesus is our best example of humility. He was God in human form but he "emptied himself," giving up all claims of the worship that should be due him. He came to earth in the form of a man, tempted to sin as all of us are, eventually to suffer for our sins. In other words, he gave up everything to be a servant. Using Jesus as our example, we too are called to empty ourselves and be servant leaders.

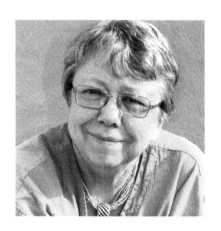

AUTHOR'S PAGE

Marja Bergen's book Riding the Roller Coaster was published in 1999, a beginning of her efforts to reduce the stigma of mental illness. Starting in the year 2000, Marja brought mental health awareness to the Christian church—a church that was still uninformed about such issues.

Her work began in earnest in 2006 with the founding of Living Room faith-based peer support groups. She saw this ministry as the most beneficial for people living with mental health challenges. It was also the most practical way for churches to serve those with mental illness. But Living Room was only part of her work.

During the next nine years she wrote a book, articles, and kept an active blog. Marja presented at several conferences, including Missions Fest, and was a guest on 100 Huntley Street. She had speaking engagements where she gave her first-person account about what it means to live with a mental illness and to have a faith that kept her strong. In addition, she was planting Living Room groups in various parts of Canada and the United States—reaching sixteen groups at one point.

Marja feels that the most important aspect of her work has been to combine faith in Christ with a seeking for mental health as a way of helping people deal with their challenges. In her mid-seventies, she continues to write and send out weekly *Reflections on Scripture* to serve this need. Most of these devotionals also appear in her weblog at www.marjabergen.com.

Marja has lived with bipolar disorder since 1965. New Life Community Church in Burnaby is currently her church home. She lives in the Vancouver area of BC, Canada with her husband Wes and has a son, Cornelius, and a daughter-in-law, Jeannette.

Printed in the USA
CPSIA information can be obtained
at www.ICGtesting.com
LVHW050814020724
784426LV00011B/170